AF734940

Garland Medieval Casebooks
Vol. 8

# MANUSCRIPT SOURCES OF MEDIEVAL MEDICINE

Garland Reference Library
of the Humanities
Vol. 1576

# Garland Medieval Casebooks

JOYCE E. SALISBURY AND CHRISTOPHER KLEINHENZ
*Series Editors*

SAGAS OF THE ICELANDERS
*A Book of Essays*
edited by John Tucker

DISCOVERING NEW WORLDS
*Essays on Medieval Exploration and Imagination*
edited by Scott D. Westrem

SEX IN THE MIDDLE AGES
*A Book of Essays*
edited by Joyce E. Salisbury

MARGERY KEMPE
*A Book of Essays*
edited by Sandra J. McEntire

THE MEDIEVAL WORLD OF NATURE
*A Book of Essays*
edited by Joyce E. Salisbury

THE CHESTER MYSTERY CYCLE
*A Casebook*
edited by Kevin J. Harty

MEDIEVAL NUMEROLOGY
*A Casebook*
edited by Robert L. Surles

SAINT AUGUSTINE THE BISHOP
*A Book of Essays*
edited by Fannie LeMoine and Christopher Kleinhenz

MANUSCRIPT SOURCES OF MEDIEVAL MEDICINE
*A Book of Essays*
edited by Margaret R. Schleissner

SOVEREIGN LADY
*Essays on Women in Middle English Literature*
edited by Muriel Whitaker

FOOD IN THE MIDDLE AGES
*A Book of Essays*
edited by Melitta Weiss Adamson

# MANUSCRIPT SOURCES OF MEDIEVAL MEDICINE

*A Book of Essays*

*edited by*

Margaret R. Schleissner

GARLAND PUBLISHING, INC.
*New York & London / 1995*

Copyright © 1995 Margaret R. Schleissner
All rights reserved

**Library of Congress Cataloging-in-Publication Data**

Manuscript sources of medieval medicine : a book of essays / edited by Margaret R. Schleissner
p. cm. — (Garland reference library of the humanities ; vol. 1576) (Garland medieval casebooks ; vol. 8)
Includes bibliographical references and index.
ISBN 0-8153-0815-9 (alk. paper)
1. Medicine, Medieval—History—Sources.
I. Schleissner, Margaret Rose. II. Series. III. Series: Garland reference library of the humanities. Garland medieval casebooks ; vol. 8.
R141.M365 1995
610'.9'02—dc20 94-15149

Printed on acid-free, 250-year-life paper
Manufactured in the United States of America

# Contents

# Acknowledgments

This project first began to take shape during two month-long research visits to the Institut für Geschichte der Medizin in Würzburg in June and October 1990. I am very grateful to the Deutsche Forschungsgemeinschaft, Sonderforschungsbereich 226 Würzburg/Eichstätt: "Wissensorganisierende und wissensvermittelnde Literatur im Mittelalter" for funding those visits and to Professor Gundolf Keil for sponsoring me. I also wish to thank Rider University for granting me a Summer Research Fellowship to prepare this volume.

I would like to thank Professor Joyce Salisbury and the editors at Garland Publishing for all their help. Above all, I owe thanks to the contributors whose efforts have made this volume possible. Finally, this book is dedicated to my husband, Richard Pelz (who contributed his computer expertise) and to my daughter, Emily.

# Introduction

The importance of manuscripts to the study of medieval medicine cannot be overestimated. Much material that is absolutely crucial to our understanding of medical thought and medical practice in the Middle Ages lies undiscovered and unedited in manuscript archives. The authors of these essays address such material from different perspectives, with different objectives, and with different results. In so doing, they uncover a number of key questions. What was the relationship between medical knowledge in written form and medical practice? How was medical knowledge produced, organized, and circulated? What do the manuscripts themselves tell us about the audience, intended or actual? What was the function and importance of vernacularization?

The majority of the essays in this volume represent substantially reworked versions of papers given in three sessions on manuscript sources of medieval medicine at the Twenty-seventh International Congress on Medieval Studies at Western Michigan University in Kalamazoo, Michigan, in May 1992. The intention of those sessions was, first, to bring to the attention of scholars in a wide range of disciplines the importance of manuscript studies in medieval medicine, and, second, to provide a forum for the exchange of ideas between European and North American historians of medieval medicine. To round out the picture, I have included two essays, not originally part of those sessions, which highlight other crucial aspects of research on medieval medical manuscripts: One on the incorporation of medical material in manuscripts pertaining primarily to another discipline (in this case, time reckoning or *computus*), and the other on the collection of medical books in medieval and early modern libraries, in this case the library of the court at Heidelberg.

The lead essay by Bernhard Schnell, "Prolegomena to a History of Medieval German Medical Literature: The Twelfth Century," stands at the beginning of the collection for two reasons. This essay not only examines the earliest manuscripts containing medical texts in German, but also it programmatically lays out methodological principles based on the latest state of manuscript research in Germany, known as *Überlieferungsgeschichte* (the study of texts from the perspective of manuscript transmission and literary sociology). Thus it comes first chronologically and it sets the tone for the entire volume. Twelfth-century medicine, it is found, is set exclusively in monasteries. That it coexists with the most up-to-date theological and philosophical writings within manuscripts, reflects a "wholistic" conception of humans that embraces their spiritual as well as physical well-being.

The essays by Gundolf Keil and Peter Murray Jones apply these principles to individual manuscripts. Keil examines in detail the background and importance of medical texts transmitted in the *Codex Berleburg*, a prime example of a medieval German *Sammelhandschrift* containing texts in Latin and German from the seven mechanical arts, including medicine. Of particular interest are the marginal annotations that span the individual segments of the manuscript (brought together in its current form by 1475), suggesting that it served as a physician's manual and was at one time used by a patient of social distinction, the Mainz canon Bernhard of Breidenbach.

Jones explores the relationship of written information to medical practice in the fifteenth century on the basis of the rare autograph evidence provided by the commonplace book of an English practitioner, Thomas Fayreford. The way Fayreford compiled the information in his commonplace book, leaving space in each category for later additions and providing guideposts such as cross-references and tables for the reader, gives us insight into the manuscript's intended use. Fayreford's manuscript contains material incorporated from other authors, as well as his own personal experience and names of practitioners and patients, bringing us, as Jones puts it, "as close as we are likely to get to the preoccupations of a fifteenth-century medical practitioner."

Melitta Weiss Adamson and William Crossgrove discuss individual works as they exist in manuscripts and early printed editions. Adamson analyzes the manuscript-tradition of Hildegard of Bingen's *Physica*, particularly with regard to five newly discovered manuscripts. Judging by the changes the text underwent in its two hundred years of manuscript transmission (1300–1500)—the selection and rearrangement of material, for example, or the translation from German to Latin and vice versa—Adamson can draw certain conclusions as to the likely audience (Latinate or German-speaking, professional or lay).

Crossgrove examines the medical material transmitted in an agricultural handbook, the *Twelve Books on Rural Practices* by Petrus de Crescentiis (or Peter of Crescent) from the early fourteenth century. The medical information that Peter considered an estate manager needed to know in order to ensure the well-being of his plants, animals, human laborers, and family members suggests a reliance on academic medicine (and bias against traditional practitioners) by the laity in the absence of academically qualified physicians.

Another text type containing medical information is the *computus*, or calendar manuscript, studied by Faith Wallis. The organization of *computus* manuscripts reflects medieval styles of education and medieval scientific mentalities. How and why medicine became associated with *computus* and what kinds of medical material these manuscripts contain are among the questions investigated by Wallis in her "reading" of the structures and contents of two manuscripts in particular.

A certain type of material found in manuscripts, namely information on birth control, is the subject of an essay by John M. Riddle. He finds evidence that classical and medieval authors knew about birth control agents (and that much of this information was added by later scribes), although they may have called them emmenagogues, drugs to promote menstruation.

The long view, leading us into the sixteenth century, is represented by Debra Stoudt's essay on the medical manuscripts assembled over time by the electoral princes in the Bibliotheca Palatina in Heidelberg. Stoudt demonstrates how the collection and preservation of medical manuscripts within libraries are dependent upon the personal health and interests of the patrons or collectors, as well as their friends and associates, their political interests, and in this case, too, the growth of university faculties. Of particular interest is the way in which the palatine electors (and Protestant German courts in general) allied themselves for political reasons with Paracelsian reformers.

Linda Voigts's essay, "Multitudes of Middle English Medical Manuscripts, or the Englishing of Science and Medicine" brings us full circle in that, like Bernhard Schnell's study of German manuscripts from an earlier period, it surveys vernacular medical manuscripts within a single national tradition. It comes at the end, also, because it treats the largest number of manuscripts and introduces a modern research tool, the *VK* (Voigts-Kurtz) database and companion volume, a supplement to the Thorndike-Kibre, *Catalogue of Incipits of Mediaeval Scientific Writings in Latin* for medieval English. Voigts's emphasis on vernacularization—its relationship to authority and its implication of new audiences—as well as on manuscripts (and the promise this major resource holds out for future scholarly work in these areas) supplies a fitting end to this collection.

The many areas of overlap among these essays—some of them very surprising—are due to the focus on manuscripts that provides the unifying theme. All essays, for example, in one way or another, illustrate the importance of manuscript transmission as a key to understanding medieval methods of organizing knowledge. What emerges from the volume as a whole is a sense of the bookishness of medieval medical culture and therefore the value of paying close attention to the primary sources. It is hoped that readers will come away with an appreciation of the richness, variety, and scope of these sources and of the vast amount of work that remains to be done. Such philological groundwork must form the foundation of future historical syntheses.

# Manuscript Sources of Medieval Medicine

# Prolegomena to a History of Medieval German Medical Literature: The Twelfth Century*

*Bernhard Schnell*

## I

The purpose of this chapter is to set out some remarks about the current state of research with regard to the history of medicine in Germany, and then, in the first main section, to say something about the methodology and the overall conception that underlie my plan to write a history of German vernacular medical literature in the Middle Ages. The second section will be concerned with an individual example, the German language medical literature of the twelfth century. These remarks about the twelfth century are to be understood as a first attempt to get a grip on the material: an essay rather than a systematic presentation. The twelfth century, with only a small number of surviving texts, would seem to be an ideal subject for such an experiment.

Anyone seeking information from the standard handbooks about the beginnings of German language medical literature—wanting to know, for example, what texts existed in the twelfth century, what literary forms are represented, by whom and for whom they were written and copied—has quite a problem.[1] A glance at any of the numerous histories of medicine that have appeared in recent years would actually suggest that there was no German medical literature at all in the Middle Ages. Neither the *Geschichte der Medizin*[2] by Erwin Ackerknecht, fifth improved and corrected edition 1986, nor Wolfgang Eckart's *Geschichte der Medizin*[3] of 1990 contains any reference to the existence of German language texts in the Middle Ages, not even to the literature on the subject. Even the new *Geschichte der Medizin*[4] by Dieter Jetter, which appeared in 1991 and by contrast with its predecessors devotes more space to Antiquity and the Middle Ages than to the modern period, is totally disappointing for our purposes. Max Neuburger's dictum of 1911, according to which German language medical literature is "predominately popular or semipopular in character" and therefore of no significance for the history of medical science, seems still to hold in the world of historical medical scholarship.[5]

In German literary studies the situation is not much better. German medical literature is seldom mentioned in literary histories. Religious and legal literature, on the other hand, has frequently been included, so it is not simply a matter of literary histories excluding texts that are not "poetic." A significant change has been brought about by the second edition of the *Verfasserlexikon*,[6] the alphabetical handbook of medieval German literature. Here for the first time, German medical texts of all kinds have been given their proper place, which is to a considerable extent the personal achievement of Gundolf Keil, as one of the principal editors and the author of the great majority of the articles. In many cases these articles have laid the first foundations for our knowledge of the texts, and it will be the task of future students of German medical history to build on the basis established by the *Verfasserlexikon*, to extend our knowledge of the transmission and sources of the German texts, and to edit the most important unpublished works. It must be borne in mind that it is a lot easier to bring corrections and modifications than to execute the original pioneering work.

## II

The fruitfulness of an approach to medieval literary studies on the basis of the transmission of texts in their manuscript copies has become increasingly apparent in recent years. The term that has come to be used to mark this approach in Germany is "der überlieferungsgeschichtliche Ansatz," the study of the history of transmission.[7] In 1983 Hans Fromm formulated this in his survey of the scholarship of German studies in the Federal Republic by saying that the approach to the study of texts and to literary history on the basis of manuscript transmission, as practised above all in the school of Kurt Ruh, could now be seen as "giving the absolute lead in historical literary research."[8] He goes on: "It is not just a matter of the astounding increase in material: the serious study of literary sociology and research into the reception of medieval literature actually are based on the study of manuscript transmission."[9]

The manuscript as a historical entity has become the starting point for the study of literature and has acquired quite new importance.[10] The individual manuscript is no longer regarded disparagingly as a more or less imperfect copy made by an incompetent scribe, and of no value in itself, but rather it has come to be seen as a prime object of study and more than simply an aid to the recovery of the author's original text. On the one hand, we have the authorial text and the author's intentions; on the other, the manuscript text and its function. Intention and function are not necessarily one. Each manuscript copy reveals the two complementary manifestations of textual transmission: on the one hand, the text itself, internal and immanent in the language of the text; on the other, the codicological context, external to the language of the text. The synthesis of these two aspects can shed light on the various gradations of textual mutation and provide new insights into medieval literary and learned culture. The methodological basis for a renewed effort to examine the German medical texts of the Middle Ages is provided by this approach that has been successfully tested on many different types of medieval texts.[11]

The starting point for my "History of Medieval German Medical Literature" must therefore be the context of the individual texts in their manuscripts. For practical reasons I am restricting myself in these prolegomena to the literature of the twelfth century. But the boundary of the year 1200 has only a paleographical basis; there is no demarcation line here in the history of literature or in the history of ideas.

Within each period the whole transmission of German medical literature needs to be documented, irrespective of whether these texts are new works or simply copies of earlier ones. Vernacular glosses on Latin texts will not be included; for the most part these have already been listed and published by Steinmeyer and Sievers.[12] Similarly individual medical recipes must in general be excluded; I am only recording those few that were written down before 1200—in view of the paucity of material surviving from this earliest period. Further areas to be excluded are veterinary medicine and most alchemical and astrological texts. In these two last categories, however, there are a number of borderline cases that have to be considered on their own merits. It is not always possible to draw a clear line between magic, charms, and witchcraft on the one hand, and medicine in the strict sense of the word on the other. When texts of this kind are associated with a healing function they will need to be included.

A preliminary examination of the material indicates that this programme will be practicable for the twelfth, the thirteenth, and probably also for the fourteenth century, although the boundaries must not be determined in advance.

It is not yet clear whether the project can be continued into the fifteenth century, which saw a huge explosion of manuscript production in Germany.

Initially the texts surviving from each period must be ordered chronologically on the basis of the manuscript transmission. Then in a second step a presentation on the basis of genre must be attempted (e.g., "medicinal handbooks," "collections of recipes," "guides to good health," and "herbals"), combined where possible with a discussion of the pragmatic context in which the texts were employed (diagnostics, therapy, prognostics, and dietetics). A subdivision of the texts according to the different medical disciplines such as anatomy, pathology, internal medicine, pharmacy, surgery, and obstetrics does not seem to be helpful with medieval texts. Such a subdivision has quite rightly been employed for later centuries by Dieter Jetter in his previously mentioned *Geschichte der Medizin*.

For the prolegomena the starting point must be the manuscripts, and in particular the dating of these manuscripts, for apart from just one or two exceptions, we have no information at all about when the texts were originally written. Many dates of composition that can be found in the literature are merely speculative, for the most part simply rough-and-ready estimates, frequently undermined by the compulsive mania that requires that every text should be as old as possible, presumably to increase its dignity. For two scholars an exception must be made: Elias Steinmeyer[13] and Friedrich Wilhelm.[14]

The method employed in most of the previous medical literature of dating the texts on the basis of the sources used is not practicable for the earliest German texts, given the present state of knowledge. Apart from Wilhelm's volume of notes[15] there is not a single study that attempts to identify the sources of the early German medical texts precisely. In any case the study of the transmission of the Latin medical texts that may have served as sources has itself scarcely begun. As long as we do not know for certain whether the presumptive source texts were actually available in the German-speaking area, it will not be possible to assemble reliable evidence that could be used for the dating of the German vernacular texts. It is not possible to assign a date on the basis of personal information about the authors of German medical literature, for in the twelfth century all the texts were anonymous.

The prospects for tackling these questions have been considerably improved in the last twenty years by the publication of manuscript catalogues and the handbooks of dated and datable manuscripts.[16] Furthermore the paleographical research of Bernhard Bischoff[17] and Karin Schneider[18] has created a more reliable basis for the dating of manuscripts. For these reasons I have elected to establish a chronology on the basis of the dating of the manuscript transmission. This at least provides reliable data about when the texts were available and when they exerted an influence. In exceptional cases in which it is possible to give a reliable date to the composition of a work, it may be possible to allow a departure from the general rule.

The procedure I am suggesting presupposes that virtually all datings of German medical manuscripts can be checked, that the manuscripts can be inspected (at least on microfilm) and—where this has not already been done—described.[19]

## III

Of the German medical texts hitherto listed in the literature, six individual works are preserved in twelfth-century copies. Ten additional manuscripts from the twelfth century contain isolated German medical recipes. The medical texts make up about 10 percent of all German vernacular manuscripts surviving from this period, whereas the greater majority of vernacular manuscripts contain poetic works and religious prose.[20]

To judge from the manuscript transmission, German vernacular medical literature begins in the second half of the twelfth century. This fits in with Hellgardt's observation that there is in general a marked quantitative increase in the transmission of German manuscripts from the second half of the century.

The beginning of German medical literature is marked by two pharmacological texts, a lapidary and a herbal: the so-called *Prüller Steinbuch* and the *Prüller Kräuterbuch*. Both of these pharmacological treatises are contained in a single codex and are conventionally named after the Benedictine monastery of Prüll in Regensburg, the earliest known provenance of the manuscript, Clm 536, (Munich, Bayerische Staatsbibliothek). The lapidary and the herbal are contained in a booklet that forms just part of the codex, in the context of a collection of shorter Latin and German medical texts.[21] This booklet is preceded in the manuscript by a series of texts that can be grouped under the heading "globus totius mundi." The most important are the *Imago mundi* of Honorius Augustodunensis, which is an encyclopedic description of the world, and the *Physiologus*, a handbook of zoological allegories, in a version that seems to have originated in France and is characterised by the omission of the chapters dealing with stones and plants. The purpose of adding the fascicle with the vernacular texts was clearly to make good this omission in the *Physiologus*. In this way the *Prüller Steinbuch* and the *Prüller Kräuterbuch*, together with a number of shorter Latin texts, are accommodated to the given context in this manuscript. It seems most likely that the individual parts of the codex were copied in Regensburg, which was one of the great centers of literary activity in the twelfth century. These first examples of *materia medica* in Germany can be dated on paleographical grounds to the beginning of the third quarter of the twelfth century. As the monastery of Prüll is recorded as having had a hospital in this period, it would have been natural to include medical texts among the books copied there.

Further copies of the *Prüller Kräuterbuch* are a fragment in Munich,[22] also from the third quarter of the twelfth century, and Innsbruck University Library Cod. 652, about which I shall have more to say later. My collation of the texts has shown that the Innsbruck manuscript was copied directly from that from Prüll. With three manuscripts, the *Prüller Kräuterbuch,* the earliest vernacular herbal in German, has to be considered one of the most widely copied German texts in the twelfth century. Only of Notker's *Psalter*, Williram's commentary on the Song of Songs, the *Kaiserchronik* (with four manuscripts and fragments), and the *Rolandslied* (also with four manuscripts and fragments) has a larger number of twelfth-century copies been preserved.

The *Prüller Steinbuch* is not, as has previously been held, a bipartite work. The text that has been described as the first part is a separate entity and consists of the beginnings of strophes one to fourteen of Bede's famous hymn *Cives superior patriae*. What Bede's hymn and the *Prüller Steinbuch* have in common is that they deal with precious stones. In Bede's Latin hymn the twelve jewels of the Heavenly Jerusalem from Revelations are described, whereas the text that truly deserves to be called the *Prüller Steinbuch* gives an account of the medicinal properties of precious stones. In this booklet, as in many other twelfth-century manuscripts, thematically associated texts are compressed together into a small space. Nevertheless, the boundaries between one text and the next are clearly marked, and the beginning of the medicinal lapidary is signalled by a bold majuscule.

The third text, the *Arzenîbuoch Ipocratis,* which belongs somewhat later in the third quarter of the century, belongs to a different genre. The earliest witness of the *Arzenîbuoch Ipocratis* is a fragment in Bamberg.[23] Only two leaves of the manuscript have been preserved, as pastedowns from the binding of a fourteenth-century manuscript of the lives of St. Clare and her sister Agnes, written in the convent of the Klarissen in Nuremberg. Nuremberg is in southeast Germany in Franconia, whereas according to Wilhelm, the dialect of the *Arzenîbuoch Ipocratis* fragment is north Rhenish-Franconian—from the valley of the Rhine—or possibly a Rhenish-Franconian copy of a south German original.

The same text is preserved in a complete copy, which Wilhelm calls the *Züricher Arzneibuch*, in a Zürich manuscript, copied in the last quarter of the twelfth century.[24] This is a manuscript of 185 leaves, all written by a single anonymous scribe. The manuscript could be described as a sort of extended florilegium. Jakob Werner, who made a detailed description of the contents in 1905, identified 391 individual texts or items, mostly Latin but with one or two German pieces and even an item in Greek.[25] The scribe has included almost the whole range of contemporary knowledge and also a number of poetical texts in German and Latin. Hexameters, elegiac distichs, and rhythmical verse forms stand alongside German and Latin prose. Werner assumes that the originator of the manuscript was a German cleric who had studied at a French university and brought this literary miscellany back with him as the fruit of his studies. Wackernagel's attribution of the manuscript to Schaffhausen and the proposal of St. Gall by Piper and Lehmann have not been confirmed by a more detailed investigation. All that can be confidently said, to use Wilhelm's formulation, is that the origin of the manuscript is to be sought somewhere in the region of Lake Constance.[26]

In addition to the *Arzenîbuoch Ipocratis*, the Bamberg fragment contains also a second German text, to which there are only occasional references in the literature. The text is important as the first example of a medical prognostic text in German, the pseudo-Hippocratic *Capsula eburnea*. It is said to have been discovered by Julius Caesar in a capsule in Hippocrates' tomb and it gives a list of the *signa mortis*, the "signs of death."[27]

The *Innsbrucker Arzneibuch* and a gynecological text entitled by Wilhelm *Frauengeheimnisse* both date from the third quarter of the century. In both cases the language is a mixture of Latin and German; both texts are preserved in the manuscript Innsbruck University Library 652, which also contains the *Prüller Kräuterbuch* mentioned above; and both texts are preserved in just this one manuscript. Like the codex from Prüll, this is a Latin miscellany with mostly theological works, containing a single booklet with a mixture of Latin and German medical literature.

Like the *Arzenîbuoch Ipocratis*, the *Innsbrucker Arzneibuch* is a collection of medical recipes organized according to the pattern *a capite ad calcem*, but the *Innsbrucker Arzneibuch* is by far the shorter of the two texts. No study of these two texts in comparison with each other has been made.

The *Frauengeheimnisse*, which begins in German but soon switches over into Latin, marks the end of the medical section of the Innsbruck manuscript. The text contains medical recipes for preparations made from animals and plants. The last sentence of the text, "audivi abbatem de superiori Scotia cum magna affirmatione dicere" ("I heard the abbot from Ireland forcefully assert"), points to the historical context in which the text was used: a monastery ruled by an Irish abbot with some experience of pharmacology. I have tried to show elsewhere that this must be Abbot Christian MacCarthy of the Schottenkloster of St. James in Regensburg.[28] At the time when this manuscript was written, St. James in Regensburg was the only monastery of Irish monks in the Bavarian dialect area. It is possible that both these texts, the *Innsbrucker Arzneibuch* and the *Frauengeheimnisse*, were written in Regensburg by an Irish monk who desired to communicate medical recipes from his homeland to his German hosts. This speculation would provide a quite new context for the assessment of the language mixture.

This brings me to the end of my survey of German medical literature in the twelfth century. What I have omitted here are the individual, isolated recipes, which would need separate treatment.

Several texts that have been claimed to be transmitted from the twelfth century are omitted from my overview: They are either not attested in twelfth-century manuscripts, as, for example, the German *Bartholomäus*, or they are transmitted in manuscripts that have been incorrectly dated, as, for example, the *Grazer Monatsregeln*.

Thus we have in the twelfth century just six German-language medical texts; their transmission is concentrated in the second half of the century and principally in the Upper German dialect area, with Regensburg as the center. The German texts are all preserved, embedded in the context of the most modern, up-to-date theological and philosophical literature in Latin: for example, Rupert of Deutz, Honorius Augustodunensis, and William of Conches. The Latin poets are represented as well: Ovid, Horace, and above all, Marbode of Rennes. The medieval medical literature in German is in this period "Mönchsmedizin." It comes from and belongs in the monasteries. Medical historians in the nineteenth and twentieth centuries have always used "Mönchsmedizin" as a derogatory term, but we must learn to understand this term in a positive sense as a precise description of the historical "Sitz im Leben" of early medieval German medicine.

When the texts are sorted as I have described, according to the date and localisation of their transmission, and their function in the historical context, the following picture emerges: Monastic medicine is embedded in a wholistic conception of man embracing both his spiritual and physical health. It is here in the monasteries that the beginnings of the scientific study of medicine can be observed and documented.[29]

## NOTES

*In honor of my teacher, Professor Dr. Hans Fromm, on 26 May 1994

1. Several essays by Gundolf Keil are first steps to remedying this situation, but they have not yet appeared in standard histories of medicine. See, e.g., "Die deutsche medizinische Literatur im Mittelalter" in: *Verhandlungen des XX. Internationalen Kongresses für Geschichte der Medizin* (Hildesheim: Georg Olms Verlagsbuchhandlung, 1968) 647–654.

2. Erwin Ackerknecht, *Geschichte der Medizin*, 5th corrected and expanded edition (Stuttgart: Ferdinand Enke Verlag, 1986).

3. Wolfgang Eckart, *Geschichte der Medizin* (Berlin, Heidelberg, and New York: Springer-Verlag, 1990).

4. Dieter Jetter, *Geschichte der Medizin* (Stuttgart and New York: Georg Thieme Verlag, 1991).

5. Max Neuburger, *Geschichte der Medizin*, 2 vols. (Stuttgart: Verlag von Ferdinand Enke, 1911) 2: 444.

6. *Die deutsche Literatur des Mittelalters: Verfasserlexikon*, founded by Wolfgang Stammler, 2nd rev. ed., ed. Kurt Ruh with Gundolf Keil, Werner Schröder, Burghart Wachinger, and Franz Josef Worstbrock, vol. 1ff. (Berlin and New York: Walter de Gruyter Verlag, 1978ff.) The following articles by Gundolf Keil are particulary relevant to this paper: "Innsbrucker (Prüler) Kräuterbuch," vol. 4, cols. 396–398; "Innsbrucker Arzneibuch," vol. 4, cols. 395–396; "Arzenibuoch Ipocratis," vol. 1, col. 505; "Prüler Steinbuch," vol. 7, cols. 875–876.

7. See, in particular, Hugo Kuhn, *Entwürfe zu einer Literatursystematik des Spätmittelalters* (Tübingen: Max Niemeyer Verlag, 1980) and the collection *Überlieferungsgeschichtliche Prosaforschung. Beiträge der Würzburger Forschergruppe zur Methode und Auswertung*, ed. Kurt Ruh, Texte und Textgeschichte 19 (Tübingen: Max Niemeyer Verlag, 1985).

8. Hans Fromm, "Germanistische Forschung in der Bundesrepublik Deutschland. Eine Umschau 1981," in *Forschung in der Bundesrepublik Deutschland*, ed. C. Schneider (Weinheim: Verlag Chemie, 1983) 113–119, here 116.

9. Fromm, 116.

10. The importance of the individual manuscript in the study of medieval German literature of all types was recognized by Gerhard Eis in his numerous studies of previously unknown texts. See, e.g., the studies reprinted in his *Forschungen zur Fachprosa* (Bern: A. Francke Verlag, 1971).

11. See, e.g., *Die 'Rechtssumme' Bruder Bertholds. Eine deutsche abecedarische Bearbeitung der 'Summa Confessorum' des Johannes von Freiberg. Synoptische Edition der Fassungen B, A und C*, ed. Georg Steer, Wolfgang Klimanek, Daniela Kuhlmann, Freimut Löser, Karl-Heiner Südekum, 4 vols., Texte und Textgeschichte 11–14 (Tübingen: Max Niemeyer Verlag, 1987) and *'Vocabularius Ex quo': Überlieferungsgeschichtliche Ausgabe*, ed. Bernhard Schnell, Hans-Jürgen Stahl, Erltraud Auer, and Reinhard Pawis together with Klaus Grubmüller, 5 vols., Texte und Textgeschichte 22–26 (Tübingen: Max Niemeyer Verlag, 1988–1989).

12. *Die althochdeutschen Glossen*, ed. Elias Steinmeyer and Eduart Sievers, 5 vols. (Berlin: Weidmannsche Buchhandlung, 1879–1923).

13. Elias Steinmeyer, *Die kleineren althochdeutschen Sprachdenkmäler*, 3rd ed. (2nd ed., 1916; repr. Berlin and Zurich: Weidmannsche Buchhandlung, 1963).

14. *Denkmäler deutscher Prosa des 11. und 12. Jahrhunderts*, ed. Friedrich Wilhelm, 2 vols. (Munich: Georg D.W. Callwey, 1914–1916).

15. Wilhelm's collection of texts consists of two parts: Part A reprints the texts; and Part B provides notes, including data about the manuscripts and sources. Many parallel texts are also printed in the notes in Part B. All the texts discussed later in my paper are included in Wilhelm's collection. They will not be individually cited in the following pages.

16. See my review of recent approaches to cataloging German manuscripts, "Überlegungen zur Katalogisierung der deutschen mittelalterlichen Handschriften," in *Zusammenhänge, Einflüsse, Wirkungen: Kongressakten zum ersten Symposium des Mediävistenverbandes in Tübingen 1984*, ed. Joerg Fichte, Karl Heinz Göller, and Bernhard Schimmelpfenning (Berlin and New York: Walter de Gruyter Verlag, 1986) 438–450.

17. Bernhard Bischoff, *Paläographie des römischen Altertums und des abendländischen Mittelalters*, 2nd ed., Grundlagen der Germanistik 24 (Berlin: Erich Schmidt Verlag, 1986).

18. Karin Schneider, *Gotische Schriften in deutscher Sprache. I. Vom späten 12. Jahrhundert bis um 1300*, 2 vols. (Wiesbaden: Ludwig Reichert Verlag, 1987).

19. I would like to thank Karin Schneider (Bayerische Staatsbibliothek, Munich) who has examined my datings of manuscripts. Ms. Schneider is widely regarded as the best qualified paleographer for evaluating medieval German manuscripts.

20. The figures on which these statements are based are taken from Ernst Hellgardt's list of Middle High German manuscripts dating before 1200: "Die deutschsprachigen Handschriften im 11. und 12. Jahrhundert. Bestand und Charakteristik im chronologischen Aufriß," in *Deutsche Handschriften 1100–1400. Oxforder Kolloquium 1985*, ed. Volker Honemann and Nigel F. Palmer (Tübingen: Max Niemeyer Verlag, 1988) 35–81.

21. See my detailed study of the *Prüller Kräuterbuch* and this manuscript: "Das '*Prüller Kräuterbuch*': Zum ersten Herbar in deutscher Sprache," *Zeitschrift für deutsches Altertum* 120 (1991): 184–202.

22. Karin Schneider, "Neue Funde frühmittelhochdeutscher Handschriftenfragmente," in *Philologische Untersuchungen. Festschrift Elfriede Stutz*, ed. Alfred Ebenbauer (Vienna: Wilhelm Braunmüller Universitäts-Verlagsbuchhandlung, 1984) 392–397, here 392–394.

23. Bamberg, Staatsbibliothek, Msc. Hist. 146 (olim E. VII. 19).

24. Zürich, Zentralbibliothek, Cod. C 58 (olim C 275).

25. Jakob Werner, *Beiträge zur Kunde der lateinischen Literatur des Mittelalters* (Aarau: H.R. Sauerländer Verlag, 1905).

26. See Werner, 1.

27. Cf. Gerhard Baader and Gundolf Keil, "Mittelalterliche Diagnostik. Ein Bericht," in *Medizinische Diagnostik in Geschichte und Gegenwart. Festschrift Heinz Goerke*, ed. Christa Habrich, Frank Marguth, and Jörg Henning Wolf (Munich: Werner Fritsch, 1978) 121–144, without this text.

28. Schnell, 1991, 199–200.

29. I wish to thank Nigel Palmer (Oxford) for translating my German text into English, for discussing the paper with me, and for providing further suggestions for improving it.

# The Textual Transmission of the *Codex Berleburg*

*Gundolf Keil*

In the area of botanical book illustration,[1] the *Codex Berleburg* must certainly be regarded as one of the most exceptional medieval German manuscripts.[2] Equally significant is the position the *Codex Berleburg* holds with respect to its textual transmission, with its remarkable number and variety of texts whose history, in some cases, extends as far back as the eighth century. In other cases, this manuscript, in the Sayn-Wittgenstein Library in Berleburg,[3] offers unique material that brings to light whole areas of crucial importance to the field of medieval German *Fachprosa*. Studying one such manuscript with a complex history of compilation can reveal much, not only about manuscript production, but about the history and transmission of the texts the manuscript contains. This essay will examine the texts of the *Codex Berleburg,* a compendium that combines medical material with texts from the seven mechanical arts, as one step in the larger process of describing the methods of compilers and the interests of users that, in turn, determine the medieval organization of knowledge.

## I. Composition

At first glance the *Codex Berleburg* appears quite complex.[4] The manuscript is considered a miscellany, because it combines several texts in a single codex. Some of the texts are in Latin[5] and some in German. In addition, it is a composite manuscript, because it holds between its covers several originally independent fascicles. The fact that different parts of the manuscript circulated independently at first is seen through the arrangement of the quires, through the fingerprints on the original first page (fol. 65r), through the arrangement in thematic units, especially the beginnings of such units,[6] and in one case, through the beginning of a new foliation.[7] Displaying the hands of more than two dozen copyists, the codex, moreover, is variously decorated, most impressively in the section on paints and dyes with its colored initials decorated in part with *fleuronné* (flower-work).[8]

Despite its complex structure, the various textual and codicological units of the *Codex Berleburg* have one thing in common: close geographical and chronological origins. The major texts were copied between 1455 and 1470, and the recipes were added later,[9] between 1475 and 1477. Geographical references point to Frankfurt am Main[10] and dialectical indicators point in the same direction. With the exception of an Alsatian scribe,[11] the dialect of all hands is Rhenish-Franconian,[12] in particular the southern variant, typical of the area around Mainz and Frankfurt.

The manuscript's contents and reception also indicate the Rhine-Main region: The surgical *materia medica* stems primarily from the recipe literature of the Upper Rhine,[13] and the numerous prescriptions are directed to a famous patient from Mainz, the canon Bernhard von Breidenbach ("bernhardus de breydenbach Canonicus maguntinus").[14] The *Codex Berleburg* also served as a direct source iconographically and textually for the *Gart der Gesundheit*[15] produced in Mainz in 1485.

Despite this geographic unity, the *Codex Berleburg* was compiled between 1455 and 1477 by various scribes with various objectives, who for the most part had only specific parts of the manuscript before them. The collection of the individual parts into a single binding occurred only at the end of the third quarter of the century, so that—as the notations which span the various segments attest—by 1475, at the latest, the *Codex Berleburg* had assumed its current composite form. In view of its complex origin, then, it is not surprising that the individual texts vary widely with respect to function, origin, age, and discipline. The texts cover several of the mechanical and occult arts and are repeated in many cases. That they ever all together formed a functional unit is highly unlikely.

## II. The Medical Texts

The most extensive complex of texts within this codex is formed by the medical texts, which represent both the oldest and the most modern texts, as well as the entire spectrum of medieval German medical literature. Most prominent among these are the two leading medical treatises of the thirteenth century, the "Elder German Macer"[16] and the "Arzneibuch" of Ortolf von Baierland.[17] To orient the reader, it is important to say a few words about the background and influence of these two texts. Both works informed medical writing in German throughout half a millennium; with the exception of the Netherlandic northwest,[18] both circulated in the entire German-speaking territory, both are transmitted in numerous manuscripts and editions, and both exhibit a complex textual history that ranges beyond the borders of German-speaking countries. Whereas Ortolf's "Arzneibuch," with over four hundred extant copies, tops the bestseller list of Middle High German literature,[19] the "Elder German Macer"—disadvantaged by various competing "Macer" translations—with over a hundred manuscript witnesses and numerous excerpts, tops the list of vernacular herbals.[20]

The "Elder German Macer" was not only retranslated into Latin, but it also underwent several adaptations, including an alphabetical reordering intended for quick reference. The *Codex Berleburg* contains various stages of this development, ranging from the original version,[21] to the reworking, to excerpts. A partial alphabetical reworking, divided into two parts and extant only in an unfinished workshop version,[22] is noteworthy because it is interspersed with additional material from the herbal of Alexander Hispanus[23] and the Thuringian "Bartholomeus,"[24] which also supplied the name "buch Bartholomei."

It should be added that the term "Macer" in medieval German medicine is just as misleading as the title "Lucidarius." Just as the German "Lucidarius" tradition[25] is only somewhat connected with the Latin "Lucidarius"[26] and the French versions[27] derived from it, so the East Central German author of the "Elder German Macer" used the eleventh-century "Macer Floridus," attributed to Odo von Meung, as his main source in addition to several other botanical-pharmacological sources.[28] His reworking includes additional antique and Salernitan sources, and divides the material into three sections: rhyme and prose prologue, herbs, and spices. Material is arranged according to botanical as well as pharmacological principles. Addressees are lay physicians; the work is dedicated to a lady who is also said to have instigated the composition. (If the work originated at the Thuringian court, this lady was perhaps St. Elisabeth; if the work arose at the court in Breslau, the patroness was likely to have been St. Hedwig.)

Traces of the ubiquitous Thuringian "Bartholomeus" can be found also in the version of Ortolfs "Arzneibuch" in the *Codex Berleburg*.[29] This Würzburg textbook of general medicine,[30] dating back to the thirteenth century, had achieved such a high level of recognition that it became useful as a model for the ordering of medical collections in general.[31] What is left of the original's highly complex system of ordering[32] in the *Codex Berleburg* is rudimentary. The Rhenish compiler was especially interested in *materia medica* for internal medicine. This caused him to further subdivide the section on internal medicine and to introduce into the various chapters (primarily therapeutic) material from other sources. Since the surgical section was missing from his Ortolf copy-text, he inserted in its place a short book of surgical recipes with a military orientation.[33] This short treatise has little thematic connection to the rest of the pieces in the compendium and thus reveals the somewhat careless nature of the Rhenish redactor's compilation. His method of compilation was not, however, entirely amateurish. Where there is no connection between the interspersed text segment and the preceding Ortolf section, there is often a thematic connection established to the subsequent group of chapters.[34]

The sources the Rhenish redactor had at his disposal reveal a wide-ranging knowledge of Latin as well as vernacular literature. A consilium for stones in the bladder,[35] for instance, is transmitted in two languages and the compiler obviously had access to vernacular texts of various dialectical origins. While the vernacular texts often appear corrupted, the Latin texts fared better. The condensed German version of the consilium for bladder stones, for example, may very well stem from the pen of the compiler. It is unlikely, however, that we are dealing with a university-educated physician and rather more likely that the redactor was a lay physician with Latin literacy.

That the Berleburg Ortolf-redactor was also not a surgeon is shown by his choice of texts, which is far too much oriented toward internal medicine. By contrast, the second text, the "Rhenish-Franconian Herbal" (see Appendix),[36] combines *materia medica* for internal diseases with surgical prescriptions taken at least in part from surgical literature of the Upper Rhine. Numerous recipes are from lay physicians—often referred to by name[37]—and the herbal itself in all likelihood was composed by a lay physician with knowledge of Latin, as is shown by the reference to his own technical incompetence and the reference to the higher technical authority of surgeons.[38] The Rhenish-Franconian dialect of the scribe suggests the Rhine-Neckar region as the origin of this compilation.

More surgical in orientation is the fourteenth text, the so-called "Berleburg Wundarznei,"[39] named after the place it is currently held rather than its place of origin. This traumatological compilation can be situated within the Mainz-Franconian region. Remedies from the "Antidotarium Nicolai"[40] and "Grabadin" of Mesuë[41] are taken from Ortolf rather than from Latin sources, especially from the final sixth treatise which balances nicely with the Berleburg Ortolf compilation, whose redactor—our Ortolf-redactor—as we have seen,[42] lacked the final surgical section of the "Arzneibuch." It is tempting to see this compiler as an apothecary who engaged in medical consultation, as was common in late medieval Germany.[43]

The "Büechelîn von guotem nutze," the eleventh text in the *Codex Berleburg*, deals primarily with internal medicine.[44] The surgical and gynecological sections exhibit a familiarity with medical literature from the Upper Rhine.[45] The treatise emphasizes prognostication, exemplified by such genres as critical days and tests for pregnancy, fertility, and recovery. An especially rare type of prognostic text is the disease-hebdomadary (a treatise on astrological disease prognostication based on the days of the week and intended for the laity), with only one other manuscript witness, which has only recently been identified as a distinct genre.[46]

Diagnostic texts are further represented in the *Codex Berleburg* by one treatise on taking the pulse,[47] two on inspection of blood,[48] and three on inspection of urine[49] (although one of these, the short treatise on urine of "Bartholomeus" appears in two separate versions).

Shortly after 1200, the Thuringian "Bartholomeus" began to disintegrate into its component parts. Complete versions are rare after 1300, and after 1400 only fragments are transmitted. Thus, in the Berleburg manuscript "Bartholomeus" excerpts are legion, not only recipes and groups of recipes but treatises. The short tract on urine from circa 1160, with which "Bartholomeus" begins, for example, appears twice in the *Codex Berleburg* in different versions.[50]

Two examples of the kinds of texts usually included in a medical vademecum are in the *Codex Berleburg*: the short treatises on phlebotomy, the "Oberdeutsches Aderlaßbüchel"[51] and the "Oberrheinisches Aderlaßbüchlein."[52] Among the other short forms of medical literature found here are the 'Regimina duodecim mensium' (regimens for health and sickness based on months of the year)[53] and the so-called wonder drug treatises (monographs dealing with a single drug of plant, animal, or mineral origin, often with magical properties),[54] whose origins range from antiquity to the late Middle Ages.

At least four[55] of the plague treatises transmitted in the *Codex Berleburg* were composed in 1349, the year the Black Death swept Germany. Two more[56] are unique to this manuscript and are likely to be just as old. A Latin plague treatise intended for Bernhard of Breidenbach is more difficult to place.[57]

The richness and variety of the recipes would be difficult to describe here. Texts on veterinary medicine and agriculture occupy a relatively small portion of the manuscript. Texts on magic, military arts, and paints and dyes, especially, are far more impressive.[58]

## III. The Annotations Concerning Bernhard of Breidenbach

In closing, a description of the annotations spanning the various parts of the manuscript is in order. All were written between 1475 and 1477. Written in various hands, all, in one way or another, relate to the one-time user of the manuscript, Bernhard von Breidenbach. That he at some time had the manuscript before him is demonstrated by entries in his own hand reflecting the entire range of interests of the manuscript itself: prevention of plague, traumatology, pharmacology, and medicinal botany, as well as textile dyes and spot removal, military technology, veterinary medicine, magic, and alchemy.[59]

Bernhard von Breidenbach was a multifaceted personality. He was at the same time a sickly man, whose pathogenic profile can be deduced from the prescriptions meant for him.[60] Nearly fifty years old, he was plagued by various respiratory, urogenital, rectal, and dermatological ailments, as well as impairment of vision. Old age and diminished libido concerned him: He took an elixir of youth, as well as external and internal sexual stimulants.

All but a few entries are written in hands other than his own. The relationship of these writers to the Mainz canon remains unknown. The variation in level of education among them is striking. Moreover, the condescending yet authoritative tone used to refer to Breidenbach: "hec breydenbach," "ille breydenbach," "idem breydenbach," and the intimate "bernhardus" together with the second-person imperatives: "nym ebben acht . . . , nit bruch es sonder noit, her breydenbach" (165va, 374v–377v, "take care . . . , do not use it unnecessarily, mister breydenbach") are address forms more suited to a physician's notebook than to the recipe collection of a patient of high social position. A recipe for an inhalant to regulate respiration which was to be administered to a patient of social distinction as requested ("dominus ipse cupit," 377r) supports the interpretation that the codex was at one time a physician's manual, as does the fact that the canon's name appears with full titles only when he names himself: *dominus bernhardus de breydenbach Canonicus maguntinus—ich Bernhardt von breydenbach Thumherre zu Meyntz* (63r, 375v).

These marginal annotations in themselves tell a dramatic story. Taken together with the medical texts transmitted in the *Codex Berleburg* they demonstrate how attention to the manuscripts themselves, the textual transmission as well as users' annotations, can tell us much about the transmission and organization of knowledge in medical *Sammelhandschriften*.

## NOTES

1. Claus Nissen, *Die Botanische Buchillustration: ihre Geschichte und Bibliographie,* 2nd ed., 2 vols. (Stuttgart: Hiersemann 1966); Felix A. Baumann, *Das Erbario Carrarese und die Bildtradition des Tractatus de herbis. Ein Beitrag zur Geschichte der Pflanzendarstellung im Übergang von Spätmittelalter zu Frührenaissance,* Berner Schriften zur Kunst 12 (Bern: Benteli, 1974); Nigel F. Palmer and Klaus Speckenbach, *Träume und Kräuter. Studien zur Petroneller 'Circa-instans'–Handschrift und zu den deutschen Traumbüchern des Mittelalters,* Pictura et poesis: Interdisziplinäre Studien zum Verhältnis von Literatur und Kunst 4 (Cologne, Vienna: Böhlau, 1990); Wolf-Dieter Müller-Jahncke, "Das Herbar des Kodex Berleburg: Entwicklung und Überlieferungs-geschichte illustrierter Herbarien . . . Die Pflanzendarstellungen des *Kodex Berleburg,*" in *Kodex Berleburg* [n. 2] 75–98, 99–105.

2. Cf. our edition: *Älterer deutscher 'Macer—Ortolf von Baierland 'Arzneibuch'—'Herbar' des Bernhard von Breidenbach—Färber–und Maler-Rezepte. Die Oberrheinische medizinische Sammelhandschrift des Kodex Berleburg: Berleburg, Fürstlich Sayn-Wittgenstein'sche Bibliothek, Cod. RT 2/6, Farbmikrofiche-Edition,* ed. Werner Dressendörfer, Gundolf Keil, Wolf-Dieter Müller-Jahncke, Codices illuminati medii aevi 13 (Munich: Edition Helga Lengenfelder, 1991).

3. Medieval town (thirteenth century) in the southern part ("Sau[d]erland") of Westphalia, Germany.

4. Cf. Werner Dressendörfer, "Kodikologische Beschreibung des Kodex Berleburg," in *Kodex Berleburg*, 7–18, 99–105.

5. Especially fols. 6ra–21va, 367r–377v.

6. Fols. 65r, 175r, 209r.

7. Fol. 268r.

8. Part 17, fols. 237va–259vb. Garlands or festoons adorn several of the initials in this section, e.g., fols. 258rb ("D"), 259rb ("N"), 259va ("N").

9. Some of these additions are dated: fols. 63r, 375r and 376r.

10. "hoc emptum anno lxxvij° in franckfordia," fol. 376r.

11. Part 3, fols. 63r–64r (war recipes).

12. Cf. Gundolf Keil, "Die Texte des 'Kodex Berleburg' im Spiegel altdeutscher Fachprosa," in *Kodex Berleburg*, 19–46, 99–105, esp. 20.

13. Cf. Gundolf Keil, *Die 'Cirurgia' Peters von Ulm. Unter–suchungen zu einem Denkmal altdeutscher Fachprosa mit kritischer Ausgabe des Textes*, Forschungen zur Geschichte der Stadt Ulm 2, (Ulm: Süddeutsche Verlagsgesellschaft, 1961); Gundolf Keil and Christian Tenner, "Das 'Darmstädter Arzneibuch.' Randnotizen zu einer oberrheinischen Sammelhandschrift der Zeitenwende," *Bibliothek und Wissenschaft* 18 (1974): 85–234; Joachim Peters, *Das 'Buch von alten Schäden. Teil I: Text*, med. Diss. Bonn 1973 [Würzburg: Königshausen & Neumann]; Ingrid Rohland, *Das 'Buch von alten Schäden. Teil II: Kommentar und Wörterverzeichnis*, Würzburger medizinhistorische Forschungen 23 (Pattensen bei Hannover: Horst Wellm Verlag [now Würzburg: Königshausen & Neumann], 1982); Dieter Lehmann, *Zwei wundärztliche Rezeptbücher des 15. Jahrhunderts vom Oberrhein. Teil I: Text und Glossar*, Würzburger medizinhistorische Forschungen 34 (Pattensen bei Hannover: Horst Wellm Verlag [now Würzburg: Königshausen & Neumann], 1985); Andrea Lehmann, *Zwei wundärztliche Rezeptbücher des 15. Jahrhunderts vom Oberrhein. Teil II: Kommentar*, Würzburger medizinhistorische Forschungen 35 (Pattensen bei Hannover: Horst Wellm Verlag [now Würzburg: Königshausen & Neumann], 1986); Jürgen Martin, *Die 'Ulmer Wundarznei.' Einleitung, Text, Glossar zu einem Denkmal deutscher Fachprosa des 15. Jahrhunderts*, Würzburger medizinhistorische Forschungen 52 (Würzburg: Königshausen & Neumann, 1991).

14. Born c. 1440, died May 5, 1497. See Dietrich Huschenbett, "Bernhard Breidenbach," in *Die Deutsche Literatur des Mittelalters:*

*Verfasserlexikon,* 2nd rev. ed., ed. Kurt Ruh with Gundolf Keil, Werner Schröder, Burghart Wachinger, and Franz Josef Woßthrock (Berlin and New York: Walter de Gruyter Verlag, 1976), vol. 1, cols. 752–754.

15. Wolf-Dieter Müller-Jahncke, "*Deßhalben ich solichs an gefangen werck vnfolkomen ließ. Das Herbar des* Codex Berleburg *als eine Vorlage des 'Gart der Gesundheit,'" Deutsche Apotheker-Zeitung* 117 (1977): 1663–1671; idem, "Das Herbar des Kodex Berleburg," in *Kodex Berleburg,* 75–98, 99–105, especially 81f.; Gundolf Keil in *Kodex Berleburg,* 71 (synonymarium of plant names); Bernhard Schnell, "Mittelalterliche Vokabularien als Quelle der Medizingeschichte: Zu den 'Synonima apotecariorum,'" *Würzburger medizinhistorische Mitteilungen* 10 (1992): 81–92.

16. William C. Crossgrove, "Macer," in *Verfasserlexikon,* vol. 5, 1985, cols. 1109–1116, esp. 1110–1112.

17. Gundolf Keil, "Ortolf von Baierland," in *Verfasserlexikon,* vol. 7, 1989, cols. 67–82.

18. The Low Countries are not completely excluded; cf. William C. Crossgrove, "'Macer'-Miszellen," in *"gelêrter der arzenîe, ouch apotêker." Beiträge zur Wissenschaftsgeschichte. Festschrift für Willem F. Daems,* ed. Gundolf Keil, Würzburger medizinhistorische Forschungen 24 (Pattensen bei Hannover: Horst Wellm Verlag [now Würzburg: Königshausen & Neumann], 1982) 403–410; *Verfasserlexikon,* vol. 7, 1989, cols. 75–77.

19. Until now, Johannes G. Mayer and I have noted 208 manuscript copies of the "Arzneibuch" and over 200 printed editions.

20. As Bernhard Schnell told me, he knows of 140 manuscripts of the "Elder German Macer"; see also *"Von den wurzen." Text- und Überlieferungsgeschichtliche Studien zur pharmakographischen deutschen Literatur des Mittelalters,* med. Habilitationsschrift Würzburg 1989, 92–177, where more than 100 manuscript copies are noted. For the competing German "Macer" translations of the Middle Ages, see 95f., and *Verfasserlexikon,* vol. 5, 1985, cols. 1112ff.; Barbara Fehringer, *Das 'Speyrer Kräuterbuch' mit den Heilpflanzen Hildegards von Bingen. Eine Studie zur mittelhochdeutschen 'Physica'-Rezeption mit kritischer Ausgabe des Textes,* Würzburger medizinhistorische Forschungen, Beiheft 2 (Würzburg: Königshausen & Neumann, 1993), passim.

21. Fols. 175ra–199rb is a complete copy of the original version.

22. Fols. 71rb–78ra, 79ra–103ra are the two parts of the Berleburg alphabetical reworking.

23. *Verfasserlexikon,* vol. 3 (1981), cols. 476–479; vol. 4 (1983), cols. 53–58; Schnell [n. 20] 230–243; Ria Jansen-Sieben, in *"ein teutsch puech machen." Ortolf-Studien,* I, ed. Gundolf Keil, Johannes G. Mayer, and

Christian Naser, Wissensliteratur im Mittelalter 11, (Wiesbaden: L. Reichert, 1993) 538–558, esp. 549f.

24. *Verfasserlexikon,* vol. 1 (1978), cols. 609–615; Gundolf Keil, "Bartholomäus," in *Lexikon des Mittelalters* (Munich and Zurich: Artemis Verlag, 1980ff.), vol. I, cols. 1498f.; Joachim Stürmer, *"von dem gîre." Untersuchungen zu einer altdeutschen Drogenmonographie des Hochmittelalters,* Mittelalterliche Wunderdrogentraktate 1, Würzburger medizinhistorische Forschungen 12 (Pattensen bei Hannover: Horst Wellm Verlag [now Würzburg: Königshausen & Neumann], 1978); idem, "Weitere Überlieferungen des mittelhochdeutschen 'Geiertraktats' sowie eine altdeutsche Übersetzung der 'Epistula vulturis,'" in *"gelêrter der arzenîe, ouch apotêker." Festschr. Daems* [n. 18] 443–478; Oskar Pausch, "Ein Zwettler 'Geiertraktat' aus dem 13. Jahrhundert," in *"gelêrter der arzenîe,"* 425–442.

25. From Marbach in southwest Germany, dating back to the end of the twelfth century; see Georg Steer, "Lucidarius," in *Verfasserlexikon,* vol. 5 (1985), cols. 939–947.

26. Ernstpeter Ruhe (ed.), *Himmel und Hölle, Heilswissen für Zisterzienser: Der 'Lucidaire en vers' des Gillebert de Cambres,* Wissensliteratur im Mittelalter 6 (Wiesbaden: L. Reichert, 1991) 68–72; see also Yves Lefèvre (ed.), *L'Elucidarium et les Lucidaires. Contribution, par l'histoire d'un texte, à l'histoire des croyances religieuses en France au moyen âge* (Paris: DeBoccard, 1954).

27. Matthias Hessenauer (ed.), *La Lumière as lais—Pierre de Peckhams Vermittlung scholastischer Theologie,* Wissensliteratur im Mittelalter 2, (Wiesbaden: L. Reichert, 1989) 41–43; Henning Düwell, *Eine altfranzösische Übersetzung des Elucidarium* (Munich: Wilhelm Fink Verlag, 1974).

28. William Crossgrove, "Zur Erforschung des 'Älteren deutschen Macer,'" *Sudhoffs Archiv* 63 (1979): 71–86.

29. Fols. 103rb–165rb (part 8); *Kodex Berleburg,* 22f., 50–54.

30. Cf. n. 19 and see Gundolf Keil, "Ortolf von Baierland," "Pseudo-Ortolfisches Frauenbüchlein," in *Verfasserlexikon,* vol. 7 (1989), cols. 67–84; Ortrun Riha, *Wissensorganisation in medizinischen Handschriften. Klassifikationskriterien und Kombinationsprinzipien bei Texten ohne Werkcharakter,* Wissensliteratur im Mittelalter 9 (Wiesbaden: L. Reichert, 1992); O. Riha, *Ortolf von Baierland und seine medizinischen Quellen. Hochschulmedizin in der Volkssprache,* Wissensliteratur im Mittelalter 10 (Wiesbaden: L. Reichert, 1992); *"ein teutsch puech machen." Ortolf-Studien, I* [n. 23]; Hans Dünninger, "Wo stand das Haus des

Mag[ister] Ortolf, 'arzet in Wirzeburc,'" *Würzburger medizinhistorische Mitteilungen* 9 (1991): 125–134.

31. It became, as Johannes G. Mayer says, a "Kompilationsleittext" (*"ein teutsch puech machen." Ortolf-Studien, I,* 54 and 57).

32. Gundolf Keil, "Zur Wirkungsgeschichte von Ortolfs Aderlaß-Kapitel ('Arzneibuch,' 73)," in *Istorgia dalla Madaschegna. Festschrift für Nikolaus Mani,* ed. Friedrun R. Hau, Gundolf Keil, Charlotte Schubert (Pattensen bei Hannover: Horst Wellm Verlag, 1985) 99–114.

33. "Kleine Wundarznei," fols. 159ra–165ra (part 8t); *Kodex Berleburg,* 22 and 53.

34. *Kodex Berleburg,* 53, and see also Dieter Lehmann and Andrea Lehmann [n. 13], vol. 2, 10–19: "Zur Gliederung von Rezeptaren," "Gliederungsprinzipien der . . . untersuchten Texte"; Johannes G. Mayer, "Zur Überlieferung des 'Elsässischen Arzneibuchs,'" *Würzburger medizinhistorische Mitteilungen* 6 (1988): 225–236.

35. Fols. 141va–142vb (part 8o); *Kodex Berleburg,* 23 and 52.

36. 'Rheinfränkisches Kräuter- und Arzneibuch' zur wunt- und lîparzenîe, fols. 6ra–21va (part 2); *Kodex Berleburg* [n. 2], 23 and 47f.

37. For example, Hertwig von Passau and Wilhelm Scheer; cf. Christine Boot, in *Verfasserlexikon,* vol. 3, cols. 1150f.; Dieter Lehmann and Andrea Lehmann [n. 13], vol. 2, 54f.

38. Fol. 14ra: ". . . vnd frege die wonden ertze wie man erkenne die fulniße [an] der farbe"; see also fol. 10ra: "diese salbe furt pellicanus in den tzyden des keysers constantini alletzydt zu stride" (*Kodex Berleburg,* 23); Werner Gerabek, "Geschichte des Pelikans: Extraktion im Mittelalter," *Zahnärztliche Mitteilungen* 81 (1991): 1498–1502.

39. Fols. 216va–237rb (part 14); *Kodex Berleburg,* 24 and 58–60.

40. Gundolf Keil, "Nicolaus Salernitanus," in *Verfasserlexikon,* vol. 6 (1987), cols. 1134–1151.

41. Gundolf Keil, "Pseudo-Mesuë," in *Verfasserlexikon,* vol. 6 (1987), cols. 451–453 and idem, "Mesuë," in *Lexikon des Mittelalters* [n. 24], vol. VI (1993), col. 567.

42. See above, p. 20.

43. Gundolf Keil, "Zur Frage der kurativ-konsiliarischen Tätigkeit des mittelalterlichen deutschen Apothekers," in *Perspektiven der Pharmaziegeschichte. Festschrift für Rudolf Schmitz,* ed. Peter Dilg with Guido Juttner, Wolf-Dieter Müller-Jahncke, and Paul U. Unschuld (Graz: Akademische Druck- u. Verlagsanstalt, 1983) 181–196; Gundolf Keil, "'meister lôrenz, des keisers apotêker.' Anmerkungen zur heilkundlichen Fachprosa des Mittelalters," in *Orbis pictus. Kultur- und*

*pharmaziehistorische Studien. Festschrift für Wolfgang-Hagen Hein,* ed. Werner Dressendörfer and Wolf-Dieter Müller-Jahncke (Frankfurt am Main: Govi-Verlag, 1985) 183–186.

44. Fols. 200va–202va (part 11); *Kodex Berleburg,* 24–26 and 54f.

45. See n. 13.

46. Fols. 201vf. ('Krankheits-Spezialhebdomadar'); see Christoph Weisser, "Mittelalterliche Wochentags-Krankheitsprognosen: Eine Gattung laienastrologisch-iatromathematischer Fachprosa," in *"gelêrter der arzenîe, ouch apotêker." Festschrift Daems,* 637–653.

47. Compare the diagnostic emphasis in the title of Ortolf's medical treatise, fol. 103rb, and see *Kodex Berleburg,* 25 and 51.

48. *Kodex Berleburg,* 25 and 42, n. 96; see Friedrich Lenhardt, *Blutschau. Untersuchungen zur Entwicklung der Hämatoskopie,* Würzburger medizinhistorische Forschungen 22 (Pattensen bei Hannover: Horst Wellm Verlag [now Würzburg: Königshausen & Neumann], 1986); Johannes G. Mayer, "Blutschau in der spätmittel-alterlichen Diagnostik. Nachträge zu Friedrich Lenhardt aus der handschriftlichen Überlieferung des 'Arzneibuchs' Ortolfs von Baierland," *Sudhoffs Archiv* 72 (1988): 225–238; Ortrun Riha, "Der Aderlaß in der mittelalterlichen *Medizin," Medizin, Gesellschaft und Geschichte* 8 (1989): 93–118.

49. *Kodex Berleburg,* 25 and 42, n. 97; Gundolf Keil, *Der 'kurze Harntraktat' des Breslauer 'Codex Salernitanus' und seine Sippe,* med. Diss. Bonn 1969; G. Keil, *Die urognostische Praxis in vor– und frühsalernitanischer Zeit,* med. Habilitationsschrift Freiburg im Breisgau 1970, 136–149.

50. Fols. 157ra–157rb (part 8s) and fols. 199rb–200va (part 10).

51. Fols. 106vb–113rb (part 8c); *Vom Einfluß der Gestirne auf die Gesundheit und den Charakter des Menschen* [Vol. I: Faksimile; Vol. II:] *Kommentar zur Faksimile-Ausgabe des Manuskriptes C 54 der Zentralbibliothek Zürich,* ed. Gundolf Keil with Friedrich Lenhardt and Christoph Weisser (Luzern: Faksimile-Verlag, 1981–1983), Vol. I, fol. 48v–55v; Vol. II, 106–120, 186f.; Friedrich Lenhardt, "Oberdeutsches Aderlaßbüchel," in *Verfasserlexikon* [n. 14], vol. 6 (1987), cols. 1274–1276; Hilde-Marie Gross, "Illustrationen in medizinischen Sammelhandschriften. Eine Auswahl anhand von Kodizes der Überlieferungs- und Wirkungsgeschichte des 'Arzneibuchs' Ortolfs von Baierland," in *"ein teutsch puech machen." Ortolf-Studien, I,* 172–348, passim.

52. Fols. 212va–216va (part 13); *Kodex Berleburg,* 26, 42 (nn. 107 and 108), 51, 56f.

53. Karin Häfner, *Studien zu den mittelniederdeutschen Zwölfmonatsregeln,* Würzburger medizinhistorische Forschungen 3 (Pattensen bei Hannover: Horst Wellm Verlag [now Würzburg: Königshausen & Neumann], 1975); Ortrun Riha, *'Meister Alexanders Monatsregeln.' Untersuchungen zu einem spätmittelalterlichen Regimen duodecim mensium mit kritischer Textausgabe,* Würzburger medizinhistorische Forschungen 30 (Pattensen bei Hannover: Horst Wellm Verlag [now Würzburg: Königshausen & Neumann], 1985); O. Riha, "Die Utrechter Monatsregeln.' Untersuchungen zur Text-geschichte," *Würzburger medizinhistorische Mitteilungen* 3 (1985): 61–76; O. Riha, "Frühmittelalterliche Monatsdiätik," *Würzburger medizin-historische Mitteilungen* 5 (1987): 371–380.

54. For example, 'Batungentraktat' (*De herba vettonica,* fol. 74rb, in part 6a); 'Eisenkrauttraktat' (*De verbena,* from "Bartholomäus") fols. 101va–102rb (in part 7c), *Kodex Berleburg,* 27 and 42f. (nn. 99 and 119); 'Kranewittbeertraktat' (Wacholderbeertraktat), fols. 102vb, 123ra, 377r (in parts 7c, 8e, 16n), *Kodex Berleburg,* 43, n. 120; 'Salbeitraktat,' fol. 374r (part 17j); 'Geiertraktat,' *Kodex Berleburg,* 59, Stürmer (1978), Stürmer (1982), Pausch [n. 24]; Rainer Möhler, *'Epistula de vulture.' Untersuchungen zu einer organotherapeutischen Drogenmonographie des Frühmittelalters,* Mittelalterliche Wunderdrogentraktate IV, Würzburger medizinhistorische Forschungen 45 (Pattensen bei Hannover: Horst Wellm Verlag [now Würzburg: Königshausen & Neumann], 1990); see also Annelore Högemann, Der altdeutsche 'Eichenmisteltraktat.' *Untersuchungen zu einer bairischen Drogen-monographie des 14. Jahrhunderts,* Mittelalterliche Wunderdrogen-traktate II, Würzburger medizinhistorische Forschungen 19 (Pattensen bei Hannover: Horst Wellm Verlag [now Würzburg: Königshausen & Neumann], 1981); Ekkehard Hlawitschka, *"wazzer der tugent, trank der jugent." Text und überlieferungsgeschichtliche Untersuchungen zum Salbeitraktat,* Mittelalterliche Wunderdrogentraktate V, Würzburger medizinhistorische Forschungen 49 (Pattensen bei Hannover: Horst Wellm Verlag [now Würzburg: Königshausen & Neumann], 1990); Sabine Kurschat-Fellinger, *Kranewitt. Untersuchungen zu den altdeutschen Übersetzungen des nordischen Wacholderbeertraktats,* Mittelalterliche Wunderdrogen-traktate III, Würzburger medizin-historische Forschungen 20 (Pattensen bei Hannover: Horst Wellm Verlag [now Würzburg: Königshausen & Neumann], 1983); Rainer Leng, "Ein lateinischer 'Kranewittbeer-Traktat' im Hausbuch Michael de Leone," *Würzburger medizinhistorische Mitteilungen* 10 (1992): 181–206.

55. Namely, the 'Schatz der wîsheit' from Straßburg (fol. 209ra–vb, part 12a); the 'Sendbrief-Aderlaßanhang' (fols. 210rb–211ra, part 12c); the plague tract of Hans von Lucken (*Kodex Berleburg,* 47 and 69); the

'Sinn der höchsten Meister von Paris' (*Kodex Berleburg,* 69); cf. *Verfasserlexikon* under these headings and Bernhard von Rostock, Heinrich von Lübeck, Heinrich von Sachsen, Rudolf Schwenninger; Hans-Peter Franke, *Der Pest-'Brief an die Frau von Plauen.' Studien zu Überlieferung und Gestaltwandel,* Mittelalterliche Pesttraktate III, 2, Würzburger medizinhistorische Forschungen 9, (Pattensen bei Hannover: Horst Wellm Verlag [now Würzburg: Königshausen & Neumann], 1977).

56. 'Ein guot lêre vür die pestilenzien,' fols. 209vb–210rb (part 12b); 'Straßburger Skabiosenwasser-Traktat,' fol. 211ra–va (part 12d); *Kodex Berleburg,* 28 and 56.

57. Fols. 374r–375r (part 17k); *Kodex Berleburg,* 72f.

58. Kodex Berleburg, 29–35.

59. *Kodex Berleburg,* 71–74.

60. *Kodex Berleburg,* 35–37.

# Appendix:
# The Texts of the *Codex Berleburg* (Summary)

1. **Short texts** (entered by various hands)

a) Inside front cover: Recipes and the plague treatise of Hans von Lucken in its Rhenish- or Mosel-Franconian version

b) 4r **Eichenmisteltraktat** and recipes for diarrhea

2. 6ra–21va **Rhenish-Franconian Herbal and Book of Medicine,** including "**Elder German Macer,**" Chs. 2, 79, and 84 (individual segments not clearly distinguished)

3. 63r–64r **Military recipe collection** in Lower Alemannic dialect (from Alsace?)

4. 65r (first page worn by constant handling) **Meister Albrant's "Roßarzneibuch"** (book of horse remedies) in the version of Siegmund von Königgrätz

5. 67va–71ra **Berleburg book of paints and dyes,** with recipes for magic, jokes, and tricks

6. [excerpted portions of a partly alphabetical reworking of the "**Elder German Macer**" (expanded from Alexander Hispanus and other sources; workshop version)]

a) 71rb–78ra [so-called "Buch Bartholomäi von der Kräuter Kraft," letter-blocks B and C (cf. note to fol. 84ra)]

b) 78rb–vb "Elder German Macer," prose prologue

7. 79ra–103ra "**Elder German Macer**": greatly expanded (partly) alphabetical version with borrowings from Alexander Hispanus and partly from the Thuringian "Bartholomeus" and its circle ('Verbena-treatise')

c) Main section: letter-blocks A, D–Z [84ra letter-blocks B and C are missing]

8. 103rb–165rb **Ortolf von Baierland,** "Arzneibuch," greatly expanded version, in part reworked into a recipe collection with "Ipocras," "Oberdeutsches Laßbüchel" and "Bartholomeus"—excerpts as well as insertions from numerous other sources

9. 175ra–199rb "**Elder German Macer**" (complete)

10. 199rb–200va **Thuringian "Bartholomeus" (Short Tract on Urine,** Paragraphs 1 and 29)

11. 200va–202va **Büechelîn von guotem nutze** (recipe collection)

12. 209ra–212va **Southwest German Compendium of Plague Treatises** (Albert of Parma, Bernhard of Rostock, Heinrich of Lübeck, Heinrich of Saxony and Rudolf Schwenninger, Straßburg **Schatz der wîsheit** of 1349)

13. 212va–216va **Oberrheinisches Aderlaßbüchlein**

14. 216va–237rb **Berleburg Wundarznei**

15. 237va–259vb **Waz du verwen wilt von sîden oder zendel** (Manual for dyers in five treatises)

16. 267v–359r **Plant names**

17. 367r–377v **(Veterinary) Medical Short Texts,** copied by various hands, including *materia medica* for Bernhard of Breidenbach by various hands, entered 1475–1477

Translated by Margaret Schleissner

# Harley MS 2558: A Fifteenth-Century Medical Commonplace Book

*Peter Murray Jones*

What use would a fifteenth-century medical practitioner have for written information? Not perhaps a question that is often asked; the best reason for this is that our own sources of information on medieval medicine are so heavily dominated by written sources. How can we know what use a medical practitioner might have made of written information if we ourselves as historians must rely on written documents alone for evidence? A leap of imagination is required. Let us imagine our practitioner for a moment as a man (though as we shall see from the manuscript discussed below, there is plenty of documentary evidence for the existence of women practitioners),[1] able to read and write both in Latin and the vernacular. Probably, therefore, he is a man who if not matriculated at a university has had some exposure to medical learning through being present in a university town with a medical faculty. He has had access to books containing medical texts and has perhaps attended lectures on the core texts of the medieval medical curriculum, the *articella*. But like many others, our medical practitioner has not necessarily taken a medical degree or obtained a license to practice. If he becomes a beneficed cleric or a friar he may well have the option to practice medicine, but will not depend on it to earn his bread. On the other hand, if for whatever reason he does not belong to one of these groups, he may depend on the practice of medicine for his living. The most profitable type of practice will be attachment to great persons at court or in the city, but it may be necessary to practice amongst lesser folk. In either case the practitioner must exploit the competitive advantages bestowed on him by the prestige of learned medicine.[2]

If he owns books then he will be able to refer to them in the course of his practice. But the evidence of surviving medical texts from a scholastic background does not suggest that, even if he is wealthy enough to own several such books, he will find them easy to use as guides to practice. Academic medical texts are admirably suited to teaching and learning, but not to the problems faced by our medical practitioner when treating patients. They are usually large and lengthy, expensive to buy, not very portable, and for quick reference purposes, difficult to look up. In Avicenna's *Canon,* for example, information about particular ailments or medicaments is scattered in different books of a very lengthy work.[3] This problem is particularly acute if our practitioner must grapple with therapeutics rather than the refined art of modification of regimen and diet to preserve complexional balance. In the matter of treatment the practitioner must in addition weigh the instruction to be gleaned from his texts against the fruits of experience, his own and that of others whom he trusts. It is not clear at all on such a hypothetical view what role written information will play in the conduct of his practice.

The survival of a manuscript which preserves the commonplace book of a fifteenth-century English practitioner named Thomas Fayreford throws welcome light on such questions. Its value as evidence is greatly increased by its having been written in the hand of the practitioner himself, rather than by a copyist. We are brought as close as possible to the mind of Thomas Fayreford when we consider this manuscript. This is not to say that we are looking here at a document meant for the private use of Fayreford alone—far from it. It is clear from the commonplace book that the compiler meant it to be of use to other medical practitioners, perhaps primarily to be of use to a son or an apprentice who would inherit the book. But by writing this text, or rather accumulation of texts, Fayreford acts as both receiver and transmitter of written information that is closely connected with the practice of medicine. The way that he compiles his commonplace book throws a great deal of light on the integration of practical experience—his own and others'—with the fruits of his own reading of medical texts. Written information is seen exceptionally to mediate medical practice rather than to act as the medium by which medical learning is preserved and transmitted within a scholastic context.

In looking closely at British Library Harley MS 2558, and in particular the part of it written in the hand of Thomas Fayreford, we will need to draw on evidence that goes well beyond what emerges from examining the textual content alone. We need to look at the mise en page and decoration of the manuscript, the order and juxtaposition of the texts, the tables and indices that guide the reader, illustrations, and cross-references within the text. Fayreford's mediating role as both receiver and transmitter of medical information required that he do more than simply act as his own scribe. The way in which he wrote different parts on different occasions, and did not proceed sequentially but by leaving space for later additions under headings already provided, has led me to call this Fayreford's commonplace book.[4] He also shaped the book in ways that would enable a reader to find his way around the text more easily and added illustrations that would supplement the information to be derived from the text. Fayreford's manuscript is a compelling reminder that a manuscript can reveal much more than the mere enumeration of texts can suggest.

But it is necessary nonetheless to start with a description of the manuscript that identifies the texts and their relationship to each other. I have adapted slightly the description provided by Tony Hunt in an earlier article on this manuscript.[5] As he says, the whole manuscript is a compendium or make-up volume, written on both parchment and paper, put together with medical interests in mind. The contents are as follows:

1. Ff. 1ra–5vb (s.xiv) Two Latin-English botanical vocabularies
2. F. 6ra/vb (s. xiv) A Latin prose passage *De osculo mulieris*, recipes *contra tussum*, an English charm, and notes on various herbs
3. Ff. 7ra–8vb (s. xiii) A bifolium containing a portion of the *Novele cirurgerie*, a versified collection of recipes in Anglo-Norman

4. F. 9r/v (s. xv) *De curis factis per T. Ffayreford in diversis locis*. A list of over one hundred named persons cured by Fayreford
5. Ff. 10ra–11vb (s. xv) A list of ailments with the name of the relevant remedial herb, beginning *Pro dolore capitis capitulo absinthium*, forming an index to the "chapters" of item 9
6. F. 12ra/b (s. xv) *Tabula super practicam scriptam post "Circa instans" in hoc volumine per Thomam Ffayreford collectam et plurimum expertam etiam experiendam Deo concedente*. This table is a guide (with medieval folio references) to item 11
7. F. 12va (s. xv) *De cirurgia collecta secundum Ffayrford*. Gives medieval folio references to cures contained in item 12
8. F. 12vb (s. xv) A short text *De saporibus et gradibus*, beginning *Novem sunt species saporum* . . . (ThK 955)
9. Ff. 13r–64v (s. xv) An alphabetical herbal, beginning *Absinthium est calidum et siccum in tertio gradu* . . . (ThK 11)
10. Ff. 65r–72r (s. xv) The *Modus medendi* of Pontius de Sancto Egidio (s. xiii) (ThK 37; this MS only)
11. Ff. 72v–124v (s. xv) *Ffayreforde* (written in gold) A medical commonplace book in Latin, with passages of Middle English, which begins deceptively with the opening lines of Roger Baron's *Practica*, beginning *Sicut ab antiquis habemus auctoribus* . . . (ThK 1479). See item 6
12. Ff. 125r–151r (s. xv) A surgical commonplace book with the rubric *Incipit Cirurgia secundum Ffayreforde*. See item 7
13. Ff. 152ra–157r (s. xiv)/157v–160va (s. xv) *Hic incipiunt judicia magistralia Egidii super urinas*, beginning *Urina nigra significat solutionem febris quartane mediante* . . . There is a section on the colour of urines (ThK 234)
14. Ff. 161r–166r (s. xiv) *De singularum egritudinum significationibus que per urinas habentes agendum est* (ThK 391; this MS only)
15. F. 166r (s. xiv) Prose passage, beginning *Omnibus horis quibus connubit homo omni muliere* . . . (ThK 993; this MS only)

16. Ff. 166v–172v (s. xiv) *Oracio pro dolore dencium* (red rubric) followed by various miscellaneous notes and blank folios. The notes seem to belong to item 11 and include (f. 169r) *Ut testatur Ysaac in libro urinarum quod quattuor sunt prime qualitates*
17. Ff. 173r–174r (s. xiv) Various medical recipes in Middle English
18. Ff. 175r–184v (s.xiv) The so-called "Letter of Hippocrates to Caesar," beginning *Ceo est la livere dy joe Ypocras enveye ay a Sesar qui joe a tey avoy promys . . .*
19. F. 185r/v (s. xiv) *Epistula a Deo de celo transmissa in Jerusalem mandatum* . . . A celebrated medieval forgery purporting to be a letter from Christ exhorting Christians to preserve the sanctity of Sunday and saints' days
20. Ff. 186r–187r (s. xiv) An anatomy, beginning *Sicut attestat .G. in Tegni volentes accedere ad phisicam primo studendum est in anathomia. Anathomia est interiorum membrorum divisio . . .* (ThK 1480)
21. F. 188ra/vb (s. xiv) Medical recipes in Latin beginning *Pro dolore dentium* (ThK 1132) and one in Anglo-Norman (f. 188vb)
22. Ff.189r-190v (s. xiv) Treatise *De aquis physicalibus*, beginning *Humana natura non minus indiget aquis physicalibus . . .* (ThK 644)
23. F. 191ra/b (s. xiv) Prognostic, beginning *Die dominica si nativitas Dei evenerit hyems bona et ventosa, estas sicca et vindemie bone . . .*
24. F. 191rb–193ra (s. xiv) Lunary, beginning *Luna prima hec dies omnibus rebus agendis utilis est*
25. F. 193ra/vb (s. xiv) A fragment (covering the letters A to C) of the *Somniale Danielis*
26. Ff. 194ra–195r (s. xiv) A medical extract from the *Secretum secretorum* with the rubric *Epistula Aristotelis ad regem Alexandrum de sanitate vite per annum*, beginning *Alexander cum sit hominis corpus corruptibile . . .* (ThK 78)
27. F. 195ra/vb (s. xiv) A set of medical charms for fevers and teeth pain

28. Ff. 197r–223v (s. xiv) Macer, *De viribus herbarum* preceded (f. 196ra/b) by a list of the herbs treated in the work together with English equivalents (ThK 610), with additional notes and names of herbs on f. 196v
29. F. 224ra/va (s. xiv) Treatise, beginning *Et quia signa lune medicinis necessaria sunt et utilia . . .* (ThK 523; this MS only)
30. Ff. 224va–225va (s. xiv) *Calendarium dieteticum* or *Dieta* attributed to Hippocrates. There is a rubric *Ego Petrus Yspanus parve scientie* and, at the end, *Explicit Tractatus magistri Petri de Yspano*
31. F. 225va/b (s. xiv) A short recipe *Ad conficiendum pillulas medicinales*
32. Ff. 226ra–227rb (s. xiv) An incomplete text of Marbod's *Liber lapidum seu de gemmis*
33. F. 227v (s. xiv) Weather prognostications. There is also a faint text, beginning *Anisum est semen feniculi . . .* which appears to be the opening of the *Synonyma Abuali* (ThK 100)

The manuscript was rebound in the 1970s, and it is unfortunate that the original binding structure was not recorded, although it is still possible to identify gatherings which have been resewn as units. There is no evidence that any of the manuscript has been added subsequent to Fayreford's ownership in the fifteenth century. The order of the manuscript has not been tampered with after Fayreford's time, nor are there any signs that text has been lost since the fifteenth century. Items 4 to 12, the second part of item 13, and some of item 16 have been written in the same hand, and as I shall explain, we can be confident that this hand is that of Fayreford himself. Items 1 to 3, the first part of 13, and the remainder of the manuscript are in a variety of hands earlier in date, and belong to the fourteenth century, or in the case of item 3, the late thirteenth century. Fayreford's hand, which can on palaeographical grounds be assigned with reasonable confidence to the first half of the fifteenth century, is also found occasionally on blank pages in the other parts of the manuscript, and he completes item 13, whose ending must have been lost. So we can assume that Fayreford inherited or acquired an assemblage of texts of earlier date, amongst which he interpolated further texts compiled by himself or copied in his own hand.

We know that Fayreford wrote these parts of the manuscript himself because of the way in which items 11 and 12 were compiled. They are compiled on what I shall call the commonplace book principle—that is to say that the compiler has allotted each heading its own share of blank paper or parchment, and then at different times added memoranda to each section beneath its heading. This can be seen from changes in the colour of the ink, and from the occasional spaces left unfilled in the text at the end of each section. It may be that a good number of medical texts were originally compiled in this way, particularly those books of practical medicine in which recipes are grouped under disease headings. Once the autograph manuscript has been copied, the signs of this method of compilation disappear, as scribes write uniformly and close up the gaps left in the exemplar. Because such fair copies (including, of course, copies of copies) survive in numbers, whereas almost all autographs of the original compiler disappear, the signs of composition on the commonplace book principle disappear too.[6] What we have in Harley MS 2558 is thus very much an exception, and all the more to be prized because of its rarity. But as a result of this manuscript evidence of compilation on the commonplace book principle, we can also be sure that items 11 and 12 in the manuscript were not copied by a scribe from an exemplar but were written by the author himself. The tables of contents to the two texts are found as items 6 and 7, and the rubrics to both tables state that the texts were "collected" by Thomas Fayreford, who is therefore both author and scribe. No copies of these texts in any other manuscript have as yet been identified.

What of the compiler, Thomas Fayreford? Unfortunately, Harley MS 2558 is almost our only source for information about him. There was a Thomas Fayreford, a Dominican named in a royal mandate as having rebelled in consequence of a direction given by the Provincial Prior after a recent visitation at Oxford in 1370, but there must be great doubt whether this is the same man despite the identical name.[7] On palaeographical grounds the parts of Harley MS 2558 attributable to Fayreford must be assigned to the first half of the fifteenth century rather than to the fourteenth. One of the cases mentioned by Fayreford in the medical commonplace text (item 11) was an apothecary treated in Oxford by Nicholas Colnet, a royal physician who accompanied Henry V on his Agincourt campaign. Colnet was a scholar of Merton College in Oxford in 1391, and became a fellow in 1398. His fellowship in Oxford was vacated in 1411, at about which time he went into royal service as clerk and physician. As Colnet became B.A. in 1395, it is unlikely that Colnet would have obtained his M.A. and subsequently the license to practise medicine before the end of the century. The case to which Fayreford alludes must have taken place at the earliest in the first decade of the fifteenth century.[8] It is therefore additionally unsafe to assume that the Dominican Fayreford at Oxford in 1370 is the same man as the compiler of the commonplace book sections of Harley MS 2558, who was most likely recalling the Colnet case in the 1420s or later.

But we can still learn quite a lot about Fayreford from his inclusion of cases of his own as well as others', cited in the commonplace book sections, and above all from the list of cures performed by Fayreford (item 4 in the manuscript). This, too, is in Fayreford's hand. In almost all of over one hundred cases (there are 103 entries on the list, but some record multiple cures), Fayreford lists the name or the place where the patient lived, or both; he also identifies the ailment or ailments, and in a few cases the method of cure. Unfortunately he gives no dates, but it is clear that the bulk of these cures were performed in Somerset and Devon, and many of the place-names (mentioned in sixty-one entries on the list) can be identified with modern places. One of his patients is named as being from Fairford in Gloucestershire, so it is likely that this was Thomas Fayreford's own place of origin, and the source of his name. Most of Fayreford's cures, however, centred on Bridgewater in Somerset, Tiverton in Devon, and the north Devon coast from Porlock in the east to Barnstaple in the west. The scattering of places named, and the way in which Fayreford refers to cures made in different places, suggest that Fayreford travelled widely in the course of his practice, presumably on horseback.[9]

We can also make some inferences about Fayreford's patients, based on the list of cures. The list of cures shows that Fayreford treated men, women, and children—sixty-three definitely male, and forty-two female, and among them seventeen children. The men are commonly named, but not the women and children, who appear usually in relation to named men. They came from several classes and social occupations. Fayreford's most important patients were Lord and Lady Poynings. Lord Poynings was presumably Robert de Poynings, Fourth Baron Poynings, born 1382, who died in 1446. Lady Poynings may have been his first wife Isabella, who died by 1434, or the second wife Margaret, who died in 1448.[10] The main family estates were in Sussex, and Fayreford may have treated them on their occasional visits to their lands in Somerset. Lady Poynings's case is first on the list and is described in more detail than most:

> Lady Poynyngs who had frenzy, and syncope and quinsy and suffocation of the womb all at once, and in three weeks she was perfectly cured with God's help.[11]

There are at least three ecclesiastics on the list, including a brother John Moles of Buckland in Devon, who appears twice. Otherwise the information on status and occupation is rather scanty. There is a miller from Tiverton in Devon, a cellarer from Bridgewater, and one "cook Geffrey," whose daughter Fayreford treated. The evidence of the list suggests that Fayreford's practice was far from being confined to people of one determinate social group, but also that, unsurprisingly, noblemen and clergy were the patients whose treatment was of most importance to him.

Given Fayreford's ability to read and write in Latin as well as in Anglo-Norman and Middle English, it seems likely that his time in Oxford—which we infer less from the appearance of a Thomas Fayreford in the university register than from his detailed description of the Colnet case—was well spent, even if he took no degree. The learning and practical experience of medicine that he picked up there must have been the basis for his successful practice in the west country. But it is also likely that Harley MS 2558 was the only medical book that he owned. Its contents include much that would be of practical benefit in diagnosis, prognosis, and therapy, and Fayreford's own interpolations suggest that his intention was that the book should be all the more useful to its next owner for the additions he made to it.

In fact, a great deal of care and expense must have gone into the additions he made to the book. The decoration is one clue—the medical commonplace book section or *Practica* (item 11) is headed at the top of the first folio by the word "Ffayreford," written in a large textura hand in gold within a cartouche. Similarly, the beginning of the herbal (item 9) is given an elaborate illuminated bar border on the top and gutter edges of the text block, and a decorated three-line initial. In all three of the main texts compiled by Fayreford himself (items 9, 11, and 12), we find rubricated initials for major sections, painted in red and blue. Fayreford himself has supplied the tiny guide letters for the rubricator to follow. Professional illuminators and rubricators must have been employed at Fayreford's expense to provide this decoration.

Fayreford has added his own foliation so that users of the manuscript can consult the tables and find the information they want in the texts he compiled. He also makes use of handy cross-references from one section in the text to another—to relate, for instance, the occurrence of syncope to suffocation of the womb, as in the case of Lady Poynings, or sometimes to save repeating recipes. Moreover, at several points in his texts Fayreford has supplied pen drawings in his own hand. Though these are informal and usually have been added outside the text block, they serve to illustrate the shape of a plaster, the appearance of an ailment, or the description of a plant. His models may well have been other contemporary English medical and surgical manuscripts, particularly those written in the vernacular, which employed decoration and marginal illustration to enhance the texts of well-known authors like Guy de Chauliac and John of Arderne (Fayreford's drawing of a patient in spasm is clearly copied from an Arderne manuscript).[12] Fayreford must have wished to emulate these authorities, and the prominence of his own name in the manuscript also suggests a conscious promotion of his own authorial fame.

In assessing the commonplace book sections of the manuscript we must not suppose that these were compiled for Fayreford's own use alone. While an entry in the commonplace book may reflect Fayreford's own reading or experience, or information he has heard from others, this does not mean that it is therefore a personal record, a memorandum made for his private use. Even the list of cures cannot be seen as a simple memorandum of cases treated, but as a means of advertising Fayreford's prowess in general, and in particular as a warrant of professional experience, evidence that Fayreford knows what he is talking about when he gives a specific remedy for a disease in the commonplace book sections.

There are three such commonplace book sections in the manuscript. The first is the herbal (item 9), which Fayreford himself misleadingly calls "Circa instans." These are the first words of a famous Salernitan herbal, which enjoyed wide currency from the thirteenth century onwards.[13] Close examination shows that Fayreford's herbal is in fact his own compilation, listing remedies for different ailments under the heading of a medicinal simple. There were gaps left at the end of the entries for each simple, allowing Fayreford and other later owners of the manuscript to make later additions. The headings are arranged in alphabetical order, but only by the first letter in the name of the herb. After each letter in the alphabet Fayreford has left a longer gap. The wide outer margins of this section of the manuscript are used for disease captions, so that a reader could see at a glance the particular ailment he was interested in within the entries for each simple.

The entry under the second heading 'arthemisia' does in fact start with very much the same formulation as the real "Circa instans," which may be why Fayreford chose to refer to this herbal misleadingly under that title. In fact the most cited authorities in the herbal seem to be the poem of Macer, *De viribus herbarum* (item 28 in this manuscript), and a commentary on the pharmacological treatise from Salerno, the *Antidotarium Nicolai.*[14] Most entries, however, are not ascribed to particular authorities, and it is not possible to tell if some of the remedies are "learned from friends or had of women" (to use the phraseology of the surgeon Lanfranc) rather than read in books. As we shall see, it is clear that the medical and surgical texts compiled by Fayreford do in fact rely on these additional sources of information.

Unlike the herbal, the two other commonplace book sections of the manuscript (items 11 and 12) are organised under the headings of different ailments. In the medical *Practica* these begin with ailments of the head and work down the body, with female ailments at the end; however, this principle of organisation breaks down increasingly, so that the last four headings are for provoking and restraining sweat, for the breasts of women, for the face, and for the giving of enemas. The surgical commonplace book makes a show of beginning with the head also, but the head to toe order breaks down even sooner. While many of the headings in the surgical section are for external and visible ailments like scabies, wounds, and apostemes, there are also headings for the stomach and for making syrups, so that it is not always clear why a particular remedy is found in this section rather than in the *Practica*. Nevertheless Fayreford includes under surgery much the same ailments as does the English surgeon John of Arderne towards the end of the fourteenth century.[15] There are indeed headings for the extraction of thorns, and for treating burns, and Fayreford obviously did not regard straightforward surgical cases like these as outside his province—there are cures for these ailments on his list, too (John Smith bitten by a dog, Thomas Mot of Fairford with a thorn in his hand).

Many of the headings in these parts of the manuscript are allocated a whole page or more, and the headings are written like running titles across the top of the first page. Ample space was left for further entries under each heading, although Fayreford ran out of space for some headings nevertheless, and had to cram his writing in as best he could by compressing the hand and using the margins. The outer margins are used to provide captions for particular remedies. This meant that the user of the manuscript could find the title of the section he wanted using the table of contents arranged under disease headings, and once he had the right section, could see from the caption in the margin the sort of remedy he wanted—perhaps a plaster, or a potion, or a charm.

Where did Fayreford get the information about remedies that he noted in the commonplace book, *Practica* and surgery? Some of it is derived from his own experience as a practitioner. There are a number of case histories which are based on Fayreford's own practical experience. A few of these can be correlated with the list of cures (item 4), as they evidently deal with the same case. For instance take the youth of Tiverton who lost the sight of his eye and recovered it with swallow's blood and betony, as the ninth item on the list of cures has it. In the section headed 'de oculis' in the *Practica* we find the following:

> There was a boy from Tiverton in Devon about twelve years of age who lost the sight of one eye after a blow to it, so that he could not see at all with the other eye closed. Twice daily I put in the affected eye swallow's blood and he drank daily betony mashed up with ale, and within fifteen days he recovered his sight by the grace of God. And certainly in many cases I have discovered betony to be effective in getting rid of all fleshy growths (?) in eyes when drunk in this fashion, and after bathing with rosewater or similar. [16]

The use of swallow's blood for eye problems is mentioned by a number of medical authorities, and probably achieved widest currency through the chapter on the swallow in the well-known encyclopaedia of Bartholomew the Englishman, *De proprietatibus rerum*, where blood from the right wing of the swallow is said to have the power of healing eyes.[17] Fayreford himself points out that the use of betony in such cases is recommended by Macer (see item 28).[18] In this way Fayreford integrated his recollections of the ailment suffered by this particular boy in Tiverton with his understanding of therapy for eye diseases based on his reading of medical authorities.

There are four other such cases in which Fayreford's relation of his cure in the commonplace book can be identified with an item on the list of cures, but in another thirty-eight cases there is no such correlation. Nevertheless, the inference in these other cases must be that Fayreford was the practitioner concerned, the hero of the story, except when he makes clear that another was involved. Some of the cases deal with named individual patients—the wife of R. le wolf, brother Iohannes de sancto egidio, and Johannes Rogge de ligtport—whom we must assume were Fayreford's patients.[19] We assume that Fayreford remembered these cases and the method of treatment he employed, and invoked them in the *Practica* to produce the warrant of previous practice in support of a particular remedy.

But the experience of other practitioners was also cited in these case histories. When Nicholas Colnet treated Hugo the apothecary in Oxford for a hectic fever complicated by jaundice, and an aposteme between liver and stomach, Fayreford may well have been there as an eyewitness—his description of this case is extraordinarily detailed. The Rector of Chesylbeck treated two cases of stomach problems, one in a male (*stomachum inflatum*) and one in a female (*stomachum in maxima dolore*), although we do not know whether Fayreford was present on either or both occasions. Other successful practitioners appear as "quedam medicus" in different cases. There are also at least two occasions when Fayreford records approvingly cases treated by females—an "amica" who treated a woman for a swollen belly with griping pain, and "quidam domina" who treated a case of sciatica in a male patient with a medicinal water when "omnes scientes in Londyn" could do nothing for him. There is a suggestion here that Fayreford was equally as happy recording the cases of unlearned female practitioners as those of university-trained physicians—so long as he thought their treatments worked.[20]

Finally there are cases that Fayreford has copied from other texts. One such is cited from Gilbertus Anglicus, involving a man stabbed with a sharp iron tool. The other seems to derive from a "magister Stephanus," who tells the story ("narrat") of a case dealing with swollen shins. It is not clear here whether Fayreford is citing a text, or which one it might be. It is even possible that Fayreford was told the story orally by Stephanus. Either way, Fayreford was willing to take the word of authority for successful cures performed by others, as well as accepting the warrant of his own experience or the evidence of his own eyes for the validity of particular remedies. The same willingness to credit authorities led him to accept recipes attributed to earlier authorities like Nicholas Tyngewick, a royal physician who died in 1339.[21] Some contemporary names cited in the text will probably only ever be known to us because Fayreford cited their names in connection with a particular recipe—magister Walter Bolle, for example, who is mentioned in several places. It would seem that word of mouth or observation of the medical practice of others played a considerable part in Fayreford's collecting of recipes. We have also to bear in mind that the citing of named authorities for particular remedies was also a means of recommending those remedies more strongly to Fayreford's audience.

Among the many recipes collected in the commonplace book were a number of *experimenta,* a term Fayreford uses to describe a recipe producing a cure but unsupported by the authority of learned medicine. Thus he talks of a remedy for 'chaudepisse': "I have heard of a wonderful *experimentum* but one that lacks any clear rationale."[22] *Experimenta* were not to be found by scanning the pages of books—or at least only by scanning pages in books like Fayreford's own collection—but typically were passed on by word of mouth, "heard," as he describes it in this instance. Most of these *experimenta* must have been heard about from other practitioners.

Most of the recipes he recommended came from earlier authors rather than from contemporary practitioners, however. The table to the *Practica* (item 6) is after all entitled "collected by Thomas Fayreford, and based both on a great deal of experience and also on what ought to be tried out God willing." What ought to be tried out is what Fayreford has based on the authority of other medical writers, some of whom are explicitly acknowledged in the text and some not. Thus the opening of the *Practica* is deceptive, since the introduction and beginning of the first section on 'dolor capitis' is a précis of the corresponding passages in the *Practica* of Roger Baron, but Fayreford goes on to add other material on "dolor capitis," and he does not make much further use of Roger Baron in the *Practica*. There is no explicit acknowledgment that this opening section is based on Roger Baron.[23] Elsewhere Fayreford is much more open about his borrowings.

His sources are not at all surprising: he uses well-known works like Bernard of Gordon's *Lilium medicine,* the compendium of Gilbertus Anglicus, John of Spain's *Thesaurus pauperum,* Guy de Chauliac, Lanfranc and John of Arderne, all of whom are acknowledged at different points. He also makes use of the Arab authorities—Avicenna, Rases, Abulcasis, Serapion, Mesuë, and others—and the standard Salernitan texts. The most quoted authorities are Gilbertus Anglicus and Bernard of Gordon, however. Whether all of these authors are quoted directly from their own works or at second hand is much harder to determine, and could probably not be settled even by an exhaustive editorial analysis. Either way, it is clear that Fayreford's reading was extensive, though probably not based on personal ownership of many medical books, given the way his own writings are integrated with the other texts in this one manuscript. His reading, if widespread, was extremely selective in its focus of interest. Almost without exception, Fayreford's compilation concentrates on therapeutics, giving very little space to description of ailments, their causes, signs, prognostication, and so on.

There are a large number of prescriptions in Middle English scattered at random through Fayreford's mainly Latin writings. These, of course, are just as likely to derive from Fayreford's reading as the Latin prescriptions, since by the first quarter of the fifteenth century there was already a considerable medical literature in Middle English, with surgery and recipe collections particularly well represented.[24] There is no real difference in kind between the Fayreford material in Latin and that in Middle English—charms, for instance, come in both languages. In Latin we are told that whoever will wear the name of Nichasius will not see spots before his eyes,[25] in Middle English, that certain sacred words must be written on the patient's cheek for toothache, and orisons said to saints Apollonia and Nichasius.[26] But it does seem as if one or two of the Middle English remedies were definitely learnt by Fayreford in the course of his travelling practice—what he titles the "operacio'"of Lady Poynings is a recipe for *demigreyne,* written in Middle English.[27] This must be the same Lady Poynings who heads the list of cures, and she must have passed on the recipe to Fayreford. Another Middle English recipe for *demigreyne* comes from a friar John, one of the white friars of London, though he may not be the original source.[28] Finally, one of the most interesting recipes is a recommendation to take a green frog that leaps in trees on sacred ground and anoint any tooth that you wish to fall out with that green substance. This curious remedy is described as "one of my secrets ('privities') that barbers have given me silver for."[29] Though Fayreford may have been a learned practitioner, he obviously did not hold himself aloof from an oral culture of secrets to be disclosed in return for silver or for favours, nor did he think that remedies deriving from this culture should be excluded from his collection, aimed as it was at an audience of other practitioners.

Fayreford's sources for the information collected in his commonplace book are various then—ranging from his own personal experience, to what he had seen or heard from other practitioners, to what he had read in the works of others. His informants were not all learned practitioners in the sense of being acquainted with Latin or Middle English medical literature, as he was himself. They included his own patients, surgeons and barbers, and women who practised medicine. By bringing all this information together in one place, grouped under convenient headings, Fayreford hoped to provide fellow practitioners with a handy guide to medical therapeutics, whether the therapy was founded on rational medical authority or consisted of *experimenta* or charms. His commonplace book is eclectic in its approach to medical knowledge and consistently pragmatic in its concentration on the efficaciousness of the remedies he copied down.

Fayreford's commonplace book writings are of exceptional rarity and significance as evidence for medical history—an example of a fifteenth-century medical practitioner digesting for his own use and that of other practitioners the information that he thought would be of most value in practice. As well as telling us incidentally a great deal about the nature of Fayreford's own medical practice, we are for once taken to the heart of the interaction of written information with medical practice. Here we see Fayreford deciding what it is that he needs to record for practical purposes—what of his own experience and what of others, what he has been told works in practice even when there is no rationale in medical theory, what he has culled from his own reading, what he has heard by word of mouth from other people. We are brought as close as we are likely to get to the preoccupations of a fifteenth-century medical practitioner.

## NOTES

1. See also Monica H. Green, "Women's Medical Practice and Health Care in Medieval Europe," *Signs: Journal of Women in Culture and Society* 14 (1988–1989): 434–473; reprinted in J. Bennett, E. Clark, J. O'Barr, B. Vilen, and S. Westphal-Wihl, eds., *Sisters and Workers in the Middle Ages* (Chicago: University of Chicago Press, 1989) 39–78.

2. On the pay of learned medical practitioners see Carole Rawcliffe, "The Profits of Practice: The Wealth and Status of Medical Men in Later Medieval England," *Social History of Medicine* 1 (1988): 61–78.

3. See the remarks of Nancy G. Siraisi, *Avicenna in Renaissance Italy. The Canon and Medical Teaching in Italian Universities After 1500* (Princeton: Princeton University Press, 1987) 21–23.

4. I mean by this the method in which the book has been compiled cumulatively over time in nonlinear fashion. I am not using the term "commonplace book" in the way that some historians of Middle English literature use it to mean the garnering of literary and practical texts in one manuscript (e.g., the Findern manuscript in Cambridge University Library), where a number of scribes and different times of writing may be involved, but there is no leaving of blank pages to be filled in later under predetermined headings. For further clarification of my specialised use of this term, see below.

5. Tony Hunt, "The 'Novele cirurgerie' in MS London, British Library Harley 2558," *Zeitschrift für Romanische Philologie* 103 (1987): 271–299. I wish to thank Tony Hunt for his kindness in allowing me to adapt his description of this manuscript for my purposes here. The notes to Dr. Hunt's article provide more detailed guidance to the texts in this manuscript than I have room for. References to ThK numbers are to columns in Lynn Thorndike and Pearl Kibre, *A Catalogue of Incipits of Mediaeval Scientific Writings in Latin*, rev. ed. (London: William Clowes & Sons, 1963).

6. For important reflections on the significance of autograph medieval manuscripts, see Gilbert Ouy, "Autographes d'auteurs

français des XIVe et XVe siècles: Leur utilité pour l'histoire intellectuelle," *Studia* Zrodłoznawcze, *Commentationes* 28 (1983): 69–103; and for a discussion of a spectrum of autographs ranging from first drafts to presentation copies, with a list of English examples, see Richard Beadle, "English Autograph Writings of the Later Middle Ages: Some Preliminaries," unpublished paper presented to the Oxford and Cambridge Seminar in the History of the Book, Cambridge, 28 October 1991. I am grateful to Dr. Beadle for allowing me to see an annotated version of this paper.

7. Alfred B. Emden, *A Biographical Register of the University of Oxford to A.D. 1500,* 3 vols. (Oxford: Clarendon Press 1957–1959) 2: 664. This Dominican Thomas Fayreford was ordained priest in 1364. There is no evidence in Harley MS 2558 for its compiler having been a priest or friar.

8. For Nicholas Colnet, see C.H. Talbot and E.A. Hammond, *The Medical Practitioners in Medieval England: A Biographical Register* (London: Wellcome Institute, 1965) 220–222.

9. This list of cures has been edited for the proceedings of a Cambridge Wellcome Unit/Consejo Superior de Investigaciones Científicas, Barcelona conference, "Practical Medicine after the Black Death," at Corpus Christi College, Cambridge, 2–5 September 1992.

10. VCH, *A History of the County of Somerset*, ed. R.W. Dunning (Oxford, 1974), vol. 3, 97, 170; GEC, *The Complete Peerage* (London, 1945), vol. 10, 663–664; *Dictionary of National Biography* (London, 1896), vol. 46, 274–275. The Poynings family of Basing, Sussex, are also possible candidates for Fayreford's patients, but the family with Somerset estates seems much more likely.

11. Harley MS 2558, fol. 9r. (All subsequent folio references are to this manuscript.)

12. Fol. 139v: on John of Arderne see n. 15.

13. See Gundolf Keil, 'Circa instans' in *Die Deutsche Literatur des Mittelalters: Verfasserlexikon*, ed. Kurt Ruh et al., vol. 1, (Berlin/New York: Walter de Gruyter, 1978) cols. 1282–1285.

14. See William C. Crossgrove, 'Macer' in *Verfasserlexikon* 5 (1985), cols. 1109–1116; Dietlinde Goltz, *Mittelalterliche Pharmazie und Medizin dargestellt an Geschichte und Inhalt des Antidotarium Nicolai, mit einem Nachdruck der Druckfassung von 1471* (Stuttgart: Wissenschaftliche Verlagsgesellschaft, 1976).

15. On Arderne see D'Arcy Power (ed.), *Treatises of Fistula in Ano, Haemorrhoids and Clysters by John Arderne*, Early English Text Society, O.S. 139 (London, 1910); and Peter Murray Jones, "Four Middle English

translations of John of Arderne," in Alastair Minnis, ed., *Latin and Vernacular: Studies in Late Medieval Manuscripts* (Woodbridge: D.S. Brewer, 1989) 61–89.

16. Fol. 78v: Erat quidam puer in etate circa xii annorum et ex percussione amisit visum unius oculi ita quod nihil potuit videre clauso alio apud tyverton in devone et inposui cotidie bis in oculo predicto sanguinem de yrundine et bibebat cotidie betonicam tritam cum servisie et infra xvnam recuperabat visum deo gracias Et certe in multis probavi betonicam esse valde evacuantem omnes ranculas sive radunculas oculorum sic potatam et lavacione aqua rosarum vel aliis.

17. Bartholomew the Englishman, *De proprietatibus rerum*, lib. 12, cap. 21. In the Strasbourg printed edition of 1505 this falls on leaf q5 verso.

18. Macer Floridus, *De Viribus Herbarum*, ed. L. Choulant (Leipzig, 1832) 46, Betonica (line 434): Non modicum prodest oculis, quos laeserit ictus.

19. Fols. 85v, 73v, 145.

20. Fols. 122v, 94v, 147.

21. Fols. 127, 145v, 99v: for Tyngewick, see Talbot and Hammond, 229.

22. Iterum audivi mirabile experimentum sed carens rationem manifestam (fol. 121v).

23. For Roger Baron see Ernest Wickersheimer, *Dictionnaire biographique des médecins en France au moyen âge* (repr. Geneva: Librairie Droz, 1979) vol. 2, 720–721, and *Supplément*, 263.

24. Rossell Hope Robbins, "Medical Manuscripts in Middle English," *Speculum* 45 (1970): 393–415; and Linda Ehrsam Voigts, "Editing Middle English Medical Texts: Needs and Issues," in *Editing Texts in the History of Science and Medicine*, ed. Trevor H. Levere (New York/London: Garland, 1982) 39–67; and L.E. Voigts and Michael R. McVaugh, *A Latin Technical Phlebotomy and Its Middle English Translation*, Transactions of the American Philosophical Society 74,2 (1984), 11–25.

25. Fol. 79.

26. Fol. 82.

27. Fol. 76.

28. Fol. 77v.

29. Fol. 82: other instances of the word 'privytes' used to describe the practitioner's secrets can be found on fols. 94v and 147.

# A Reevaluation of Saint Hildegard's *Physica* in Light of the Latest Manuscript Finds

*Melitta Weiss Adamson*

In recent years Hildegard of Bingen's work has been studied, edited, and translated by an ever increasing number of scholars from various fields. In 1979, the year which marked the 800th anniversary of her death, Hildegard was commemorated and celebrated in Germany and all over Europe. In Switzerland the *Basler Hildegard-Gesellschaft* was founded with the goal of making her work accessible to a wider audience through cheap reprints of earlier editions,[1] new translations of the texts,[2] and a vast secondary literature on Hildegard, which is now available in German, French, Italian, English, and Flemish.[3] In addition, the society publishes a journal, the *Hildegard-Zeitschrift*,[4] which appears several times a year, and it markets a wide range of Hildegard products including health food, drugs, books, records, shoes, bedspreads, precious and semiprecious stones, and woodenware.[5] In 1990, the "Friends of Hildegard" launched a fund-raising campaign that was to enable them to rent the castle of Königsegg from the municipality of Reichenau on Lake Constance, and adapt it as a Hildegard-retreat, where visitors could experience a Hildegard-lifestyle complete with spelt-cuisine, medical treatments, concerts, seminars, and meditative dance.[6]

Of particular importance for my topic, the manuscript tradition of Hildegard's *Physica*, is an unusual contest that the society started in 1984: It set a prize of five thousand Swiss francs for the first new manuscript of the *Physica* or *Causae et Curae* to be discovered.[7] This action, combined with an already steadily rising interest in and familiarity with Hildegard's medical work, led to the discovery of four new manuscripts of the *Physica* in the 1980s, and the rediscovery of one manuscript of which Hildegard scholars had been unaware for some time. The existence of five additional manuscripts is all the more stunning if one considers that until 1956 only a total of three manuscripts of the *Physica* was known to Hildegard scholars: Cod. 6952 of the Bibliothèque Nationale in Paris, written between 1425 and 1450, which formed the basis for the nineteenth-century edition by Daremberg and Reuss in Migne's *Patrologia Latina* series; Cod. Guelf. 56. 2, Aug. 4° of the Herzog-August-Bibliothek in Wolfenbüttel, written in the late thirteenth or early fourteenth century; and Cod. 2551 of the Bibliothèque Royale in Brussels, written around 1450.[8]

In 1956, Marianne Schrader and Adelgundis Führkötter added to this list a fifteenth-century fragment of the *Physica* contained in Cod. 525 (fols. 18r–23r) of the Burger Bibliothek in Bern.[9] The codex, which consists of compilations from the areas of medicine and science, was once owned by a "Doctor barbatus" from Bern, who lived in the second half of the fifteenth century.[10] The Bern fragment was included by Christel Meier in the second edition of the *Verfasserlexikon*,[11] and consulted by Marie-Louise Portmann for her new German translation of the *Physica* in six volumes, which was published between 1982 and 1984.[12]

In 1983 scholars learnt of a manuscript find of the *Physica* in Ms. laur. Ashb. 1323 of the Biblioteca Medicea Laurenziana in Florence, written around 1300.[13] According to Raimund Struck, it was Dom C. Lambot from the Abbey of Maredsous who pointed the parchment codex out to Father Dr. Petrus Becker from the Abbey of St. Matthias in Trier, who in turn identified it as the *Physica* of Hildegard of Bingen. Apart from the fact that it is one of the two oldest versions of the text we now have, the codex is remarkable for the information it contains on such aspects as ownership and price. Written around 1300 in the Rhineland, the volume was owned in the fourteenth century by a surgeon named Wydonius, who in 1385 sold it to another surgeon, Wilhelmus de Riet, for "6 florenis." Another owner was the Villmar branch of the Abbey of St. Matthias in Trier. More recently, presumably during Napoleonic times, the codex was in the collection of the Frenchman J.B. Huzard. Before the middle of the nineteenth century it was bought by Professor Wilhelm Libri, whose collection was acquired by Lord Ashburnham in 1847. In 1884, part of the Ashburnham collection was incorporated into the Biblioteca Medicea Laurenziana, where the codex is still housed today.

Around the same time the Florence manuscript became known, Raimund Struck was working in Marburg on a critical edition of one segment of Hildegard's *Physica*, the book on stones ("Liber lapidum"). As his basic text, he initially used the Wolfenbüttel version, and later a newly discovered fragment contained in Cod. 178a of the Universitätsbibliothek in Freiburg, written in the early fifteenth century.[14] When he learnt of the Florence manuscript, he soon switched to it as his leading manuscript, since its lapidary turned out to be more complete than that in the other versions.[15] Struck published his edition in 1985, unaware of another complete *Physica*–manuscript, whose discovery was announced in the *Hildegard-Zeitschrift* in 1986. The text is contained in Cod. Ferraioli 921 of the Biblioteca Apostolica Vaticana in Rome, written at the end of the fourteenth or beginning of the fifteenth century.[16] Ursula Heierle from the *Hildegard-Gesellschaft* came across the manuscript in the Vatican while acting on the assumption that copies of Hildegard's writings had been sent to Rome at the time of her canonization process.

At approximately the same time, I was able to identify parts of the *Kochbuch Meister Eberhards* as being excerpts from the *Physica*.[17] The cookbook is found in Cod. Oettingen-Wallerstein III 1, 2° fol. 43, which dates back to the last quarter of the fifteenth century, and is now housed in the Universitätsbibliothek Augsburg.[18]

As for the recently rediscovered manuscript, it was known to scholars as early as 1862, when Carl Jessen reported on a codex containing the introduction and most of Book I ("De herbis") of the *Physica* in German translation.[19] The manuscript is

Ms. germ. fol. 817 (fols. 2r–61v) of the Staatsbibliothek Preußischer Kulturbesitz in Berlin, which was written in Speyer in 1456 by a certain Wilhelm Gralap.[20] In the early 1940s, a typescript of the herbal, also known as the *Speyrer Kräuterbuch*, ended up at the Institut für Geschichte der Medizin in Würzburg, where Gundolf Keil identified it as a transcription of the Berlin manuscript. An edition of the herbal, which in addition to the *Physica* includes excerpts from the Latin and German *Macer floridus* and the *Circa instans*, is currently being prepared by Barbara Fehringer.[21] Regrettably, the manuscript eluded both Engelbert Krebs and Christel Meier in their respective articles on Hildegard in the first and second edition of the *Verfasserlexikon*.[22]

All in all, we now know of nine manuscripts, five of the complete *Physica*, of which two go back to approximately 1300, and four fragments from the fifteenth century. The number of known manuscripts has thus increased dramatically over the last decade, and yet, the only "modern" edition accessible to scholars is over a hundred years old, based on one fifteenth-century manuscript only, and complemented with passages from the first printed edition published by J. Schott in Strasbourg in 1533.[23] A new edition of the *Physica* which takes into consideration all extant Latin and vernacular manuscripts is badly needed.[24] In this chapter, I will take a closer look at the individual manuscripts, especially the ones that were recently discovered, to try and determine which one comes closest to the archetype and should be used as the leading manuscript of a future critical edition, as well as the changes the text underwent in two hundred years of transmission, from circa 1300 to 1500. Some remarks on who the compilers, translators, and users were that turned to Hildegard's medical work as a source of information and inspiration will conclude this preliminary survey.

Although we may never know what the *Physica* looked like in its original form, since no manuscript has come down to us from the first 150 years of its existence,[25] we can nevertheless get a sense of what the archetype may have been by comparing all the extant manuscripts and identifying the one that is most complete and contains material from all of the sometimes quite disparate versions. The text that best meets these criteria appears to be the Florence manuscript, one of the recent discoveries, which was copied around 1300. It contains a prologue, nine books dealing with plants, elements, trees, stones, fish, birds, animals, reptiles, and metals, as well as a list of synonyms. Indications of the drugs are provided in the margins throughout the manuscript and listed again at the end.[26] The Wolfenbüttel version, which at first glance appears equally complete, missing only the list of indications, is clearly inferior to the Florence manuscript due to its many gaps. For the book on stones, Raimund Struck has noted that sometimes the Wolfenbüttel text even breaks off in the middle of a sentence, which led him to believe that either the source used by the scribe was corrupt or the scribe himself was, as Struck put it, extremely absentminded.[27] To illustrate just how much the Florence and Wolfenbüttel manuscripts at times differ from one another, I have chosen the section on cinnamon in the respective manuscripts:

> Cod. Guelf. 56.2, Aug. 4 , fol. 9r
> Capitulum XX.
> Cynamomum etiam valde calidum est et fortes habet vires et etiam modicam humiditatem in se tenet. Sed calor eius tam fortis est quod humiditatem illam deprimit. et qui eum sepe comedit malos humores in eo minuit ac bonos humores in eo parat.
>
> [Cinnamon is also very hot, has strong powers, and holds in itself a moderate amount of humidity . . . , but its heat is so strong that it suppresses that humidity. And he who eats it often reduces the bad humors in himself, and it creates good humors in him.]
>
> Ms. laur. Ashb. 1323, fol. 4vb
> Cinamomum etiam valde calidum est. et fortes vires habet. et etiam modicam humiditatem in se tenet. sed calor eius tam fortis est. quod humiditatem illam deprimit. et qui eum sepe comedit malos humores in eo minuit. ac bonos humores in eo parat.
> Arbor cuius cortex cinamomum est valde calida est et medicinis apta unde homo qui a gutta paralisis fatigatur et qui coctidias [quotidianas] ter[tianas] quar[tanas] habet vas calibe factum tollat et in illud vinum bonum fundat. et

> de ligna et foliis prefate arboris dum succum in se habent imponat. et ad ignem fervere faciat et calidum sepe bibat. et sanabitur. nam vis eiusdem succi cum calore vini temperata et in calibineo vase cuius vis febribus resistit excocta et sic in potu sumpta quamlibet paralisim atque alias febres bonis viribus suis et temperamentorum aut additorum consumit.
> Et homo cui caput gravatum et obtusum est ita quod flatum per nares difficulter emittit et introrsum trahit cinamomum pulverizet et eumdem pulverem cum bucella panis sepe comedat aut in manu sua lingat et noxios humores per quos caput obtusum est dissolvit per virtutem caloris et temperamentum fortitudinis sue.
>
> [. . . The tree whose bark cinnamon is, is very hot and suitable for drugs. And a man who is fatigued by guttural paralysis and who has one, three and four-day fever, should take a vessel made of steel and pour in it good wine, and put in it the aforesaid wood and leaves of the tree when they have sap in them. And he should bring it to a boil on the fire and drink it often hot and he will be healed. Since the strength of this sap, tempered with the heat of the wine, cooked in a steel vessel whose strength resists the fevers, and drunk in such a potion, consumes the paralysis and other fevers with its good strengths, temperaments and others.
> And a man whose head is heavy and stuffed such that he emits the mucus through his nose only with difficulty and draws it back inside, should pulverize cinnamon and should eat this powder often with a morsel of bread or should lick it in his hand and it dissolves the noxious humors through which the head is stuffed by virtue of the heat and temperament of its strength.]

While the Wolfenbüttel version gives only the general description of the humoral qualities of cinnamon, the Florence text also discusses the medicinal properties of the cinnamon tree, and provides recipes for cinnamon potions and powders. The streamlined fifteenth-century versions which contain the section, all seem to follow the shorter Wolfenbüttel text.[28] In fact, not until the 1533 printed edition of the *Physica* does the additional material on cinnamon reappear, which suggests that Schott had access to a fairly complete manuscript in the tradition of the

Florence text.[29] It would be a mistake, however, to dismiss the Wolfenbüttel text simply as an abridged version of the Florence manuscript, comparable to the fifteenth-century examples. In the section on nutmeg, for instance, which immediately follows that on cinnamon, the descriptions are equally complete in both the Wolfenbüttel and Florence codex,[30] while the fifteenth-century versions have reduced the text to the first paragraph. Not surprisingly, it is again the sixteenth-century print which contains the entire treatise.[31] Despite its "erratic nature," the Wolfenbüttel manuscript offers valuable assistance in reconstructing the archetype: Overall the text is not very corrupt, has fewer abbreviations, and is in general easier to decipher than the Florence version.

The different treatment of the indications and Latin synonyms of the drugs in the extant manuscripts of the *Physica* gives the impression that this information was not part of the archetype, but constitutes attempts by a later audience to turn Hildegard's description of nature into a text suitable for medical practice. If this is the case, then the Wolfenbüttel manuscript has to be regarded as the representative of a later stage in the work's transmission than the Florence manuscript. The indications, which in the Florence codex are found in the margins, have become part of the main body of text in the Wolfenbüttel version, and the Latin terminology provided in the list of synonyms at the end of both manuscripts, has also replaced most of the German terminology, especially in the first book of the Wolfenbüttel *Physica,* where German plant names at the beginning of numerous sections are crossed out and their Latin equivalents are provided in the margins.[32] The trend towards substituting German *termini* with Latin ones is even more pronounced in the fifteenth- and sixteenth-century versions. But compilers/scribes were not always sure whether they chose the correct term, as illustrated in the section on "Blutwurtz" in the Bern fragment, which bears the heading "Credo quod sit tormentilla."[33] The confusion of the compiler/scribe is understandable if one considers that in the Middle Ages the name "Blutwurtz" was used for a variety of plants, as Irmgard Müller points out:

> Als "blutwurz" bzw. lateinisch "sanginaria" wurden in Mittelalter verschiedene. Pflanzen mit blutstillenden Eigenschaften bezeichnet, vor allem das Hirtentäschelkraut Capsella bursa-pastoris (L.) Meidk, sowie der hiermit vielfach verwechselte Vogelknöterich Polygonum aviculare L., insbesondere aber die noch heute als Blutwurz bekannte Potentilla erecta.[34]
>
> [In the Middle Ages various plants with styptic qualities were called bloodwort or Latin "sanguinaria," especially shepherd's pouch Capsella bursa-pastoris (L.) Meidk, as well as knotgrass Polygonum aviculare L., but mainly Potentilla erecta, still known today as bloodwort.]

Other substitutions in the Bern fragment include "Enula" for "Alant," "Fungus" for "Hirtzswam," "Aquilegia" for "Cranchsnabel," "Aristologia" for "Byverwurtz," "Serpillum" for "Quenula," "Lappa" for "Cletta," and "Pyrus" for "Birnbaum."[35] In the Augsburg fragment "Hecht" is replaced by the Latin "Lucius,"[36] and in the Freiburg fragment the German verb "krymet" is replaced by "comprimit."[37] In some cases the reasons for substituting German terms with Latin ones may have been aesthetic, as in the Freiburg quote, but mainly they appear to have been practical. The trend towards standardizing the *materia medica* and thereby giving preference to the Latin terminology in vernacular translations as well, can be observed in many fifteenth- and sixteenth-century medical works, such as the herbal of Ortolf von Baierland and the *Elder German Macer*.[38] The *Speyrer Kräuterbuch*, which contains major portions of the *Physica* in German translation, is yet another example of this phenomenon. Although the entire herbal is in German, the plants are listed in alphabetical order under their Latin names. At the beginning of each section their German equivalents are given. Hence we read: "Arthimesija heisset biboß oder buckel," or "Abrothanum heißt gertwurtz oder stabwurtz," or "Absintheum heisset wermuet" [Arthimesija is called mugwort, or Abrothanum is called southernwood, or Absintheum is called wormwood].[39]

The Vatican and Paris manuscripts of the complete *Physica*, both of which date back to approximately the first half of the fifteenth century, are very similar in style and content. Although plants, elements, trees, stones, fish, birds, animals, reptiles, and metals are all dealt with in the Vatican codex, the elements are not numbered separately, which is why the scribe only counts eight books. Major irregularities occur in the list of fish, where the individual sections are given random numbers or, at times, no numbers at all, and the contents of fol. 45r and 45v appear in reverse order.[40] Similarly, fol. 1r and 1v have been switched, which is why the treatise begins with the end of the prologue (fol. 1r) and the list of the first 82 plants of Book I, followed by the beginning of the prologue (fol. 1v) and the remaining list of plants (fol. 2r–v). As in the Wolfenbüttel manuscript, the indications of the drugs appear as subheadings in the main text. The slightly more streamlined Paris manuscript does not contain any subheadings; this may indicate that the source used by the two scribes—if in fact it was the same one—was a manuscript that provided the indications in the margins, similar to the Florence codex, thus prompting two very different editorial decisions: integration of the marginal glosses on the one hand, and their omission on the other. A more recent editorial decision worth mentioning in this context was made by Daremberg and Reuss in the nineteenth century: Their edition of the Paris manuscript does not include the German appendix (fols. 232v–238v) which constitutes a highly abridged version of parts of the *Physica*, predominantly the plants. This unique appendix, not found in any of the other extant manuscripts of the work, is written in the same hand as the Latin treatise, and includes indications in Latin either as part of the text or in the margins.[41]

According to Raimund Struck, the "Nicolaus Guglerus" named on fol. 1r as one of the owners of the Paris codex, was a sixteenth-century physician and bibliophile from Speyer.[42] Since the Berlin manuscript that contains excerpts from the *Physica* in German translation was written in Speyer (see above), the question arises whether the Paris manuscript was the actual source for the *Speyrer Kräuterbuch*. A comparison of selected passages from the two versions shows that the German translation in the herbal follows almost verbatim the Latin text of the Paris codex, and does not contain any additional material found in other manuscripts of the *Physica*, which would seem to support this hypothesis.[43]

Of the three complete *Physica* manuscripts from the fifteenth century, the Brussels version stands out as being the one with the highest degree of scribal intervention. While it contains most of the material found in the nine books of the other manuscripts, the order in which the items appear is often significantly different. There are indications that the tables of contents at the beginning of the various books were put together after the text had been copied, so as to reflect the new arrangement.[44] The page references given in these tables are in letter-form (aa, ab, ac, . . . , ba, bb, bc, etc.), which corresponds with the pagination system used for the codex as a whole. Overall the material has been shifted around more in the first half of the manuscript (i.e., the books on plants, elements, and trees) than in the second half. Fish, birds, and animals are treated in an order almost identical to that in the other manuscripts. Following the general trend of replacing Hildegard's German terminology with a Latin one, the Brussels manuscript goes farther than the other versions, and reduces the amount of German in the text to a bare minimum.

Apart from the formal changes of rearrangement and translation, the substance of the *Physica* has been altered through omissions and additions to such a degree that the Brussels manuscript could almost be regarded as an original compilation. Raimund Struck's observation that many magic formulas are missing from the book on stones, but on the other hand material has been added that shows strong similarities with other lapidaries, holds true for the remaining books of the *Physica* as well.[45] Time and again the compiler/scribe has pruned out passages referring to magic in favor of more "scientific" explanations.[46] Little wonder then that mandrake, the plant which throughout the Middle Ages was synonymous with magic, is completely missing from the Brussels text. Among the additional sections are "bitumen" (fol. 33r), "Medo," "Claretum," "Pigmentum," and "Cera" (fol. 35r), "Sicamorus" (fol. 44r), "Pellicanus" (fol. 85r–v), "Dromedarus" (fol. 96r), and "Sulphur" (fol. 118v). In numerous instances the information provided by Hildegard has been complemented with excerpts from other works.[47] In the section on "Laurus" the compiler/scribe has even been found to add gradus information to Hildegard's description of the plant's humoral qualities (fol. 41v).[48] As in the Florence manuscript, the indications of the drugs appear in the margins. Furthermore, the Brussels version lists a number of Latin and German synonyms for plants and animals in the individual tables of contents, as well as in the margins of the main text.[49]

This brief analysis of the Brussels manuscript makes clear that its compiler/scribe was well-versed in Latin medical and technical literature, and may even have been university-trained. His changes to the style and substance of Hildegard's work were obviously attempts to "modernize" the *Physica* and bring it up to the level of fifteenth-century science and technology. Many times the supernatural is suppressed in favor of the rational and, judging from the additions, the compiler/scribe had considerable expertise in the areas of chemistry and metallurgy.[50]

Of the fifteenth-century fragments of Hildegard's work, only one, the Freiburg manuscript, forms a homogeneous entity in that it constitutes the copy of one entire book of the *Physica*: "De lapidibus." Written around 1400, the Freiburg lapidary shows strong similarities with the Florence manuscript.[51] Since the book on stones is not included in the 1533 printed edition of an otherwise remarkably complete manuscript in the Florence tradition (see above), Raimund Struck surmised that the Freiburg fragment may be the missing part of the very manuscript which Schott used as his source.[52] However, unless the latter surfaces one day, it will be next to impossible to substantiate Struck's claim.[53] Scribal intervention in the Freiburg text is minimal, and as in the Florence manuscript, the indications of the drugs are provided in the margins.

In the Bern fragment the interventions of the compiler/scribe are similar to those observed in the Brussels manuscript, and include additions, omissions, rearrangement, and translation. What follows after the title "Hyldegardis de simplicibus medicinis" is a hodgepodge of approximately thirty chapters, only nineteen of which I was able to identify as being excerpts from the *Physica:* sixteen from Book I, "De plantis"; and three from Book III, "De arboribus."[54] After thirteen sections copied from Hildegard, the compiler/scribe begins to insert material from other sources that often complements the information contained in the *Physica*. Hence the tree "savina," the first item discussed in the Bern fragment (fol. 18r), is dealt with again in the middle of the treatise (fol. 20r), and in the appendix (fol. 22v), which is written in the same hand as the main text, only in smaller script. The plant "enula," item two in the manuscript, also reappears in the appendix (fol. 22r–v). Since the Bern codex contains a number of herbals, such as the *Tractatus medicus de plantarum vi* (fols. 18r–133v), *Macer de herbis* (fols. 134r–166v), *Herbarius* (fols. 172r–181v), and *De viribus herbarum [Serapionis]* (fols. 210r–334v), it is likely that the additional information was derived from one or several of these sources.[55]

The *Physica* material in the Bern manuscript represents a selection and rearrangement of individual simples taken primarily from three areas of the book on plants: sections 29 to 35, 95 to 98, and 144 to 172 in the *Patrologia Latina* edition (see note 54), which may be an indication that the compiler/scribe only had access to portions of Hildegard's work. As in the Brussels manuscript, the Middle High German terms have largely been replaced by Latin ones, although in several instances the original German term is also provided. This is the case with "Fvngus qui dicitur hirszswam" [Fungus which is called "Hirschschwamm"](fol. 18r), "Aquilegia id est krancsnabel" [Aquilegia that is cranesbill] (fol. 18v), "Aristologia vel rustica id est biuerwurtz" [Aristologia or rustica that is "biuerwurtz"] (fol. 18v), and "Lappa haec quae cletta dicitur" [Lappa which is called bur thistle] (fol. 22r).

In the Bern fragment of the *Physica* the indications of the drugs are integrated in the text, and short references to them appear in the margins, such as "vermes," "pulmo," and "fungus" (fol. 18r). The appendix, which was compiled from other sources, does not contain any marginal glosses.[56]

While the Bern codex seems to have been put together for a medical practitioner with a good command of Latin and a strong interest in pharmacology, the Augsburg codex gives the impression that it was compiled for a much broader and primarily German-speaking audience. It belongs to a type of composite manuscript known as "Buch vom Menschen, Tier und

Garten," which usually contained a pharmacopoeia or a *Regimen sanitatis*, a book of horse remedies, and a book on grafting.[57] With its pharmacopoeia ("Arzneibuch," fols. 2r–58v), cookbook ("Das Kochbuch Meister Eberhards," fols. 59r–70r), book of horse remedies ("Meister Albrants Roßarzneibuch," fols. 73r–79r), and book of ointments and plasters ("Salbenbuch," fols. 79v–83v), the Augsburg codex varies only slightly from the norm. The codex is written in one hand, and frequently alternates between German and Latin, especially in the pharmacopoeia and the cookbook. The book of horse remedies contains only a small number of Latin insertions, and the recipes for ointments and plasters are all given in German.[58]

When Anita Feyl edited the *Eberhard*-cookbook in 1963, she omitted nearly all the Latin passages in the text, which is one of the reasons why Hildegard's authorship remained undetected for so long.[59] The cookbook is made up of three parts: culinary recipes (fols. 59r–60v), a dietetic list of foodstuffs (fols. 60v–69r), and medicinal oils (fols. 69r–70r). The first time the compiler quotes the *Physica* is at the end of the culinary section. His goose recipe (fol. 60r–v) is the Middle High German translation of a major portion of Hildegard's chapter "De ansere" in Book VI of the *Physica*, "De avibus."[60] The rest of the Hildegard material appears in Latin and is incorporated in the dietetic list of foodstuffs. It encompasses nearly all of Book V, "De piscibus," ten of the first eleven chapters of Book I, "De plantis," and three more chapters of Book VI, "De avibus."[61] The compiler thus had access to at least three books of the *Physica*.

On the whole, the Hildegard excerpts constitute a shorter and more concise version compared to the other manuscripts. On the level of style the interventions of the compiler/scribe, who was obviously fluent in German and Latin, extend beyond rearrangement and translation. Syntax and vocabulary are also frequently changed, whereby for instance the noun "slim," the Middle High German term for phlegm, at times appears in its adjectival form "sleymig."[62]

With the discovery of Hildegard's *Physica* as one of the sources for the cookbook, we now know practically all the works of medieval *Fachliteratur* from which the treatise was compiled. The type of material and the way it was selected, arranged, and translated in the manuscript suggest a compiler who had a good command of Latin but was unlikely to have received his education at any of the major medical schools of the time. The cookbook combines medical-dietetic literature from three different periods and geographic areas: Hildegard's *Physica,* written in Germany, reflects monastic medicine that does not yet bear the stamp of Arabism; the *Breslauer Arzneibuch,* from which he extracted the section on medicinal oils, is rooted in the *Corpus Constantinum,* and hence is a product of the school of Salerno;[63] while most of the dietetic list of foodstuffs was copied from the pseudo-Arnaldian *Regel der Gesundheit,*[64] which in turn is a translation of Konrad von Eichstätt's enormously popular *Regimen sanitatis,* in particular the treatise "De qualitatibus ciborum."[65] Konrad based his regimen on works by Avicenna, Rhazes, and Averroës, which were part of the *Corpus Toletanum,* and were used as textbooks at the medical schools of Montpellier and Paris.[66] The culinary recipes at the beginning of the cookbook show strong similarities with other German recipe collections of the fourteenth and fifteenth centuries, above all the *Buoch von guoter spîse.*[67]

In his 1969 dissertation on the *Secretum secretorum,* Wolfgang Hirth suggests the Cistercian Abbey of Seligenthal in Landshut as a likely place for the compilation of the codex. He points to the fact that the "Herzog Heinrich" mentioned in the title of the *Eberhard*-cookbook was one of the Abbey's benefactors, and that physicians, scribes, and cooks are listed among the lay people employed by the Cistercian nuns of Seligenthal.[68] This kind of environment would explain the good working knowledge of Latin that the compiler of the codex displays, and the inclusion of such texts as Hildegard's *Physica,* which could be found in monastic libraries and private collections, but never became part of medieval school medicine. For his study, Hirth was primarily interested in the first treatise of the Augsburg codex, the "Arzneibuch" (fols. 2r–58v), which contains excerpts from the *Secretum secretorum* in German translation. Among the other sources for the "Arzneibuch" identified by Hirth are the *Praktik des Meisters Bartholomäus,* the *Macer Floridus,* the *Arzneibuch Ortolfs von Baierland,* and a *Branntweintraktat.*[69] Not mentioned by Hirth or Karin Schneider in her recent description of the codex is the *Regimen sanitatis Salernitanum*, whose Latin verses are interspersed throughout the *Arzneibuch*.[70] A reference to Platearius (fol. 11v) points to the *Circa instans* as another source the compiler may have used.[71] Composite manuscripts put together from the works listed above and miscellaneous smaller treatises were not uncommon in the late Middle Ages. They, in fact, formed a standard corpus of monastic medicine of which many examples have survived.[72]

From his analysis of the *Secretum*-excerpts in the *Arzneibuch*, Hirth concluded that the compiler had access to a Latin and a German version of the encyclopedia, but instead of simply copying the German source, he chose, for the most part, to create an independent translation which closely followed the Latin text.[73] As in the cookbook, some Latin passages have remained untranslated. In one instance, a mistake made by the translator may be seen as an indication that his qualities as a cook surpassed his qualities as a translator: The *Secretum*-passage "lactuce agrestes" ("wild lettuce") appears as "laktuken vnd agreste" ("lettuce and 'agreste'") in the Augsburg manuscript (fol. 2r). For the Latin adjective "agrestis" the German noun "agreste" is given, which incidentally is the standard culinary term for a sour sauce made from unripe grapes and other unripe fruit.[74]

The similar compilation method applied in the cookbook and the *Arzneibuch*, and the expertise in nutrition also apparent in the *Arzneibuch*, strongly suggest one and the same compiler for both texts,[75] a compiler who could be assumed to have drawn on Hildegard for his pharmacopoeia as well. My examination of the *Arzneibuch* revealed that this was indeed the case. I have so far been able to identify a total of fifteen chapters, eight dealing with plants and seven others with trees, which were extracted from the *Physica* and incorporated in two areas of the *Arzneibuch*, described by Karin Schneider as "Rezeptsammlung, dt. und lat." and "Heilpflanzen. dt. und lat."[76] The *Physica*-excerpts appear in the order "Alant," "Feniculum," and "Tille" (fol. 8v), "Item der pawm der wachalterenn ist" (fol. 10v), "Vom Rettich" (fol. 11v), "Vonn Benedicten wurtz" (fol. 12r), "Die Lorber" (fol. 29r), "Item Vom kutenpawm," "Item Eyban pawm," "Item Enula," "Item Birca" (fol. 48r), "Item hauswurtz," "Item fennu grecum" (fol.

48v), "Item Tylia" (fol. 48v), and "Item Tormentilla" (fol. 52r).[77] I was surprised to find that the amount of German is much higher in these Hildegard passages than the ones included in the cookbook, where only the goose recipe is given in translation. With the exception of "Feniculum," all the excerpts in the *Arzneibuch* are in German, and only occasionally a Latin sentence or phrase is interspersed in the text.

With the *Physica* as the link between the *Arzneibuch* and the cookbook, it is almost certain that both were compiled by the same individual who had access to Hildegard's book on trees, in addition to the books on plants, fish, and birds that he used as a source for the cookbook. Why the compiler chose to translate some but not all of the *Physica*-excerpts into German is not entirely clear. He may have set out to write the whole codex in German, but capitulated whenever the Latin became too difficult to translate.[78] By the time he put together the cookbook, he may have found even this method too tedious, and decided to simply copy the Latin text of his source. The fact that the cookbook is generally more structured than the *Arzneibuch*, may be regarded as another sign that the compiler knew more about cooking and nutrition than about pharmacology.

In the *Arzneibuch* of the Augsburg codex, no attempts are made to synthesize the information on herbs derived from the *Macer Floridus, Elder German Macer, Physica,* and other works, and to arrange all the material in alphabetical order. This degree of synthesis is, however, achieved in the Berlin manuscript that is compiled from much the same sources as the *Arzneibuch*: the *Macer Floridus, Elder German Macer, Physica,* and *Circa instans*.[79] The Berlin herbal begins with a German translation of the preface to Book I of Hildegard's *Physica*, which is followed by the rhymed and prose prologues to the *Elder German Macer* (fols. 1r–3r). Although the herbs are listed in alphabetical order under their Latin names, the compiler also provides one or more German synonyms for a given plant at the beginning of each chapter. The thrust of the material is copied from the *Elder German Macer*, and complemented with passages from the *Macer Floridus* in German translation. The *Physica*-excerpts are all in German and usually appear at the end of a chapter. This is the compilation method used, for instance, for the herbs

"Arthimesija," "Abrothanum," and "Absintheum" (fols. 3r–5r). The information on "Archangelica" is derived solely from the *Macer Floridus*, while the chapter on "Allium" is based on the *Elder German Macer*, and the *Macer Floridus* (fols. 5r–6r).[80]

Unlike the *Arzneibuch* in the Augsburg codex, the *Speyrer Kräuterbuch* is written entirely in German. A comparison of the German Hildegard passages in both manuscripts shows that they constitute two independent translations of the Latin text.[81] Given that in the Berlin manuscript the *Physica* is integrated in a herbal, it should not surprise us to find that the excerpts are taken from Hildegard's book on plants, a book which occupies more than one third of the entire work. The Berlin fragment is thus not just the most extensive German translation of the *Physica* that has come down to us, but also the most extensive of all four fragments. Together with the German excerpts in the Paris and Augsburg manuscripts it bears witness to a well-established vernacular tradition of Hildegard's medical work in the fifteenth century.

When in 1857 the Paris manuscript of the *Physica*, the only one known at the time, was published, many scholars became acquainted with the work, and this in turn led to the discovery of three new manuscripts.[82] With scholarship initially focusing on complete manuscripts and the reconstruction of the archetype, vernacular versions such as the appendix to the Paris manuscript and the Berlin fragment were neither edited nor studied in any detail—and were eventually forgotten. It was not until 1956 that Schrader and Führkötter reported on another manuscript find, the Bern fragment. Since it was part of a larger medical compendium, they suspected that more *Physica*-manuscripts were likely to be discovered once the vast medical literature of the Middle Ages was properly catalogued and analyzed.[83] History certainly proved Schrader and Führkötter right: The enormous interest in recent years in medieval *Fachliteratur* in general, and Hildegard's medical writings in particular, culminated in the discovery of two complete *Physica*-manuscripts, two fragments, and the rediscovery of a third fragment. With the exception of the Vatican version, all the new manuscripts have one thing in common: They make no reference to the actual author or title of the work, on the contrary, as illustrated by the title "lapidarius ysydori" of the Freiburg fragment (fol. 1r), which for nearly six hundred years fooled librarians into thinking that they were dealing with a lapidary by Isidore of Seville.

The transmission of the *Physica* from the thirteenth to the fifteenth centuries, as evidenced in the nine extant manuscripts, shows numerous attempts on the part of the audience to make the text more "user-friendly." Indications of the drugs and lists of synonyms were added. Hildegard's German terminology for the *materia medica* was gradually replaced by Latin, while on the other hand her Latin prose was increasingly translated into the vernacular. By studying the context in which the manuscripts, and here in particular the fragments, appear, we can gain insights into which books of the *Physica* had the widest appeal. The book most often excerpted, rearranged, and translated in the fifteenth century was undoubtedly Book I, "De plantis." With its more than two hundred foodstuffs and drugs, it was at times treated as a herbal in its own right, to be copied either separately or in conjunction with other herbals such as the *Macer Floridus* and *Circa instans*. It is followed in popularity by the *Physica's* Book III, "De arboribus"; Book IV, "De lapidibus"; Book V, "De piscibus"; and Book VI, "De avibus."

Although every new manuscript find of a medieval work adds to our knowledge of the text and its history, I would argue that three of the recently (re-)discovered *Physica*-manuscripts are more important than the others, namely: the Florence manuscript, which is closest to the archetype and will play a pivotal role in any future critical edition; the Augsburg fragment, with the valuable insights it provides into the work of a fifteenth-century compiler and translator; and the Berlin manuscript, which to date constitutes the most extensive German translation of the *Physica* and the first complete integration of Hildegard's book on plants into a herbal.

# NOTES

1. The reprints include the *Patrologia Latina* editions of the *Physica* (repr. Basel: Basler Hildegard-Gesellschaft, 1982) and *Liber Divinorum Operum* (repr. Basel: Basler Hildegard-Gesellschaft, 1983) included in J.P. Migne, ed. *S. Hildegardis Abbatissae Opera Omnia* (Paris: Garnier, 1882), cols. 739–1036, and cols. 1117–1352; and Paul Kaiser, ed., *Hildegardis Causae et Curae* (Leipzig: Teubner, 1903; repr. Basel: Basler Hildegard-Gesellschaft, 1980).

2. Marie Louise Portmann, trans., *Heilmittel: Deutsche Übersetzung der Physica mit Berücksichtigung aller Handschriften*, 6 vols. (Basel: Basler Hildegard-Gesellschaft, 1982–1984).

3. For a complete list of Hildegard literature see Hildegard-Vertriebs AG, *Preisliste für Hildegard–Mittel und Reformprodukte* (March 1989) 17–20.

4. *Hildegard-Zeitschrift* 1 (1981).

5. See *Preisliste für Hildegard–Mittel*, 3–23.

6. See promotional material "Ein Schloss für Hildegard" sent to members of the *Internationale Gesellschaft Hildegard von Bingen* in 1990.

7. The contest is announced in Portmann, *Heilmittel*, 5: 2.

8. For the dating of the three manuscripts see Raimund Struck, "Hildegardis De Lapidibus Ex Libro Simplicis Medicinae: Kritische Edition unter Vergleich anderer Lapidarien," med. diss. Marburg, 1985, XXI, XXVII, XXVIII.

9. Marianne Schrader and Adelgundis Führkötter, *Die Echtheit des Schrifttums der Heiligen Hildegard von Bingen* (Cologne/Graz: Böhlau, 1956) 56; for a description of the codex see Hermann Hagen, *Catalogus Codicum Bernensium (Bibliotheca Bongarsiana)* (Bern: Haller, 1875) 439f.

10. Schrader and Führkötter, *Die Echtheit des Schrifttums*, 56, n. 47.

11. Christel Meier, "Hildegard von Bingen," in *Die Deutsche Literatur des Mittelalters: Verfasserlexikon*, eds. Kurt Ruh, Gundolf Keil, Werner Schröder, Burghart Wachinger, and Franz Josef Worstbrock. (Berlin/New York: Walter de Gruyter, 1981) vol. 3, col. 1272.

12. See Portmann, *Heilmittel*, 4: 188.

13. For the dating and history of the parchment codex see Struck, "Hildegardis De Lapidibus," XI.

14. For the dating and description of the fragment see Struck, "Hildegardis De Lapidibus," XVIIf.

15. See text-critical comments in Struck, "Hildegardis De Lapidibus," 88.

16. For the dating and description of the manuscript see *Hildegard-Zeitschrift* 5 (1986): 21–23.

17. Melitta Weiss-Amer, "Die 'Physica' Hildegards von Bingen als Quelle für das 'Kochbuch Meister Eberhards,'" *Sudhoffs Archiv* 76 (1992): 87–96.

18. For the dating and description of the codex see Karin Schneider, *Deutsche mittelalterliche Handschriften der Universitätsbibliothek Augsburg: Die Signaturengruppen Cod.I.3* and *Cod.III.1* (Wiesbaden: Otto Harrassowitz, 1988) 234–238.

19. Carl Jessen, "Über Ausgaben und Handschriften der medizinisch-naturhistorischen Werke der heiligen Hildegard," in *Sitzungsberichte der Mathematisch-Naturwissenschaftlichen Classe der Kaiserlichen Akademie der Wissenschaften*, [Vienna], 1. Abtheilung, 45 (1862) 97–116, esp. 111–113.

20. William Crossgrove, "Zur Erforschung des 'Älteren deutschen Macer,'" *Sudhoffs Archiv* 63 (1979) 77f.

21. I wish to thank Dr. Gundolf Keil for informing me about the manuscript, and Barbara Fehringer for sending me excerpts of her dissertation on the *Speyrer Kräuterbuch*.

22. See Engelbert Krebs, "Hildegard von Bingen," in *Die Deutsche Literatur des Mittelalters: Verfasserlexikon*, ed. Wolfgang Stammler, vol. 2 (Berlin/Leipzig: Walter de Gruyter, 1936), col. 443; and Christel Meier, "Hildegard von Bingen," *Verfasserlexikon*, 2nd ed., vol. 3, col. 1272.

23. The complete title of the Strasbourg edition is *Physica S Hildegardis Elementorum, fluminum aliquot Germaniae, metallorum leguminum fructuum et herbarum: arborum et arbustorum: piscium denique volatilium et animantium terrae naturas et operationes IIII libris mirabili experientia posteritati tradens*. Argentorati. J. Schott 1533. According to Carl Jessen, the 1544 edition of the *Physica* is merely a reprint of Schott's version under a different title; see Jessen, "Über Ausgaben und Handschriften," 97f.

24. In 1982 Professor Irmgard Müller announced that she was embarking on a critical edition of the *Physica;* however, it is not known how far she has progressed in her work since then; see Irmgard Müller, *Die pflanzlichen Heilmittel bei Hildegard von Bingen* (Salzburg: Otto Müller Verlag, 1982) 19, n. 15.

25. The *Physica* is presumed to have been written between 1151 and 1158; see Sabina Flanagan, *Hildegard of Bingen, 1098–1179: A*

*Visionary Life* (London and New York: Routledge, 1989) 225; 1150–1157 are the dates given in Engelbert Krebs, "Hildegard von Bingen," col. 448.

26. The contents of the Florence manuscript are as follows: fol. 1r Prologus, fols. 1r–28r de herbis, fols. 29r–31r de elementis, fols. 31r–48v de arboribus, fols. 48v–59v de lapidibus, fols. 59v–68v de piscibus, fols. 68v–80v de avibus, fols. 80v–93v de animalibus, fols. 93v–97v de vermibus venenosis, fols. 97v–99r de metallis, fols. 99v–100r Synonyma Lat. and Ger., fols. 100r–101r Varia medicinalia, fols. 101r–104r List of indications, fol. 104v Varia (entries by different hands).

27. See Struck, "Hildegardis De Lapidibus," 88, 91; the contents of the Wolfenbüttel manuscript are as follows: fol. 1r–1v Prologus, fols. 2r–62r de herbis, fols. 62v–66v de elementis, fols. 67r–90r de arboribus, fols. 90r–106v de lapidibus preciosis, fols. 106v–120r de piscibus, fols. 120r–140v de volatilibus, fols. 141r–162r de animalibus, fols. 162r–168v de vermibus, fols. 168v–173r de metallis, fols. 173r–174v Synonyma Lat. and Ger.

28. Paris manuscript PL. col. 1139; Vatican manuscript fol. 4rb; the section is missing in the Brussels manuscript.

29. In his comparison of the Wolfenbüttel codex with the Paris manuscript and Strasbourg edition, Hermann Fischer lists numerous instances in which the printed edition contains substantially more material than the Wolfenbüttel text; see Hermann Fischer, *Die Heilige Hildegard von Bingen, die Erste Deutsche Naturforscherin und Ärztin: Ihr Leben und Werk* (Munich: Verlag der Münchner Drucke, 1927) 113–158.

30. In the printed edition the additional text runs as follows:

> *De arbore cinnamomi*. Arbor cujus cortex cinnamomum est valde calida est. Unde homo qui a gutta paralysis fatigatur, et qui quotidianas, tertianas, et quartanas habet, vas de chalybe factum tollat, et in illud bonum vinum fundat, et de ligno et foliis praefatae arboris, dum succum in se habent, imponat, et ad ignem fervere faciat, et calidum saepe bibat, et sanabitur. Et homo cui caput gravatum et obtusum est, ita quod flatum per nares difficulter emittit et introrsum trahit, cinnamomum pulverizet, et eumdem pulverem cum buccella panis saepe comedat, aut in manu sua lingat, et noxios humores per quos caput obtusum est, dissolvit. (PL, col. 1139, n. 3)

31. Compare the versions Florence fols. 4vb–5ra, Wolfenbüttel fols. 9r–10r, Paris PL, col. 1139, Vatican fol. 4rb–va, and PL, cols. 1139–40, n. 5, for the additional material in the Strasbourg edition; the section is missing from the Brussels manuscript.

32. The Middle High German terms are crossed out in red ink, while brown ink is used for the Latin terms provided in the margins in very small script; see Struck, "Hildegardis De Lapidibus," XXI. It is not clear when these substitutions were made.

33. Bern, Burger Bibliothek, Cod. 525, fol. 19r.

34. Irmgard Müller, *Die pflanzlichen Heilmittel*, 54.

35. See Bern manuscript, fols. 18r, 18v, 22r, 20v; and PL I 95, 34, 144, 146, 98; and III 2.

36. Augsburg manuscript, fol. 64r; PL V 9.

37. Freiburg manuscript, fol. 10ra; PL IV 13; see also critical edition in Struck, "Hildegardis De Lapidibus," 54.

38. James Follan, *Das Arzneibuch Ortolfs von Baierland* (Stuttgart: Metzler, 1963); Crossgrove, "Zur Erforschung des 'Älteren deutschen Macer,'" 71–86, esp. 76f.; William Crossgrove and Bernhard Schnell are currently preparing an edition of the *Elder German Macer*.

39. These quotes are taken from Barbara Fehringer's preliminary transcription of the Berlin manuscript.

40. Whether the irregularities are due to scribal error or mistakes in collating cannot be determined at this point; the reverse order of some pages of the book would seem to indicate the latter, however.

41. See Struck, "Hildegardis De Lapidibus," XXV.

42. Struck, XXIII.

43. Compare, e.g., *Arthimesija*, *Abrothanum*, and *Absintheum* in the Berlin manuscript (fols. 3r–5r) with their counterparts *Stagwurtz*, *Biboz*, and *Wermuda* in PL I 106, 107, 109 (cols. 1171–1173); Carl Jessen also found that the excerpts in the Berlin manuscript correspond exactly with those in the Paris text. His qualification that in some "rare" cases additional material showed similarities with Schott's printed edition, is not backed up by any concrete evidence; see Jessen, "Über Ausgaben und Handschriften," 112.

44. An example is the plant "Binsuga," which is missing from the table of contents of Book I; the scribe may have overlooked the section when he listed the various items because the initial "B" was never completed in the main text (fol. 17r).

45. See Struck, "Hildegardis De Lapidibus," 90f.

46. Compare, e.g., fols. 39r–54v ("De arboribus") with PL III, cols. 1215–1248.

47. See esp. the metals on fols. 114v–118v and their counterparts in PL IX, cols. 1345–1350.

48. Hildegard does not include gradus information, i.e., levels of intensity, when she describes the basic qualities hot, cold, wet, and dry; for the history of the gradus system see Georg Harig, *Bestimmung der Intensität im medizinischen System Galens* (Berlin: Akademie-Verlag, 1974), esp. 195–203.

49. See the contents of "De herbis" on fol. 4r, or fol. 19r, where *Beynwelle* is given in the margins for the Latin *Consolida*.

50. His background may have been similar to that of Conrad Kyeser, who in his monumental work on medieval warfare entitled *Bellifortis*, demonstrates a profound knowledge of the Latin language, technology, and medicine; see Conrad Kyeser aus Eichstätt, *Bellifortis*, ed. and trans. by Götz Quarg (Düsseldorf: Verlag des Vereins Deutscher Ingenieure, 1967) 19–25.

51. Struck, "Hildegardis De Lapidibus," 90.

52. Struck, X.

53. According to Schrader and Führkötter, a certain Canon Bruno who had close ties to the Rupertsberg monastery, may have copied both of Hildegard's medical works and subsequently taken them to Strasbourg; see Schrader and Führkötter, *Die Echtheit des Schrifttums*, 55, esp. n. 46; also Fischer, *Die Heilige Hildegard von Bingen*, 29f.

54. They correspond with PL I 29, 30, 32, 34, 35, 95, 98, 144, 145, 150, 151, 162, 166, 172, and III 2, 21, 23.

55. For a complete description of the codex see Hagen, *Catalogus Codicum Bernensium*, 439f.

56. Only one comment, "Per contrarium," is found in the margins of the appendix (fol. 22v); it refers to an underlined passage in the section on *savina* describing the plant's abortive qualities.

57. As to the genre and its variations, see Anita Feyl, "Das Kochbuch Meister Eberhards: Ein Beitrag zur altdeutschen Fachliteratur," diss. Freiburg, 1963, 9–12; also Wolfgang Hirth, "Studien zu den Gesundheitslehren des sogenannten 'Secretum Secretorum': Unter besonderer Berücksichtigung der Prosaüberlieferungen," diss. Heidelberg, 1969, 27f.; and Birgit Zimmermann, "Das Hausarzneibuch: Ein Beitrag zur Untersuchung laienmedizinischer Fachliteratur des 16. Jahrhunderts unter besonderer Berücksichtigung ihres humanmedizinisch-pharmazeutischen Inhalts," diss. Marburg, 1975.

58. A detailed description of the Augsburg codex is included in Feyl, "Das Kochbuch Meister Eberhards," 1–4.

59. As to the discovery of the *Physica*-fragment see Weiss-Amer, "Die 'Physica' Hildegards von Bingen," 91.

60. Feyl, "Das Kochbuch Meister Eberhards," 90f., recipe 24; in PL VI 10, col. 1293.

61. See concordance in Weiss-Amer, "Die 'Physica' Hildegards von Bingen," 91f.

62. A comparison of selected passages in the *Eberhard*-cookbook with their counterparts in PL is found in Weiss-Amer, "Die 'Physica' Hildegards von Bingen," 92–94.

63. See C. Külz and E. Külz-Trosse, *Das Breslauer Arzneibuch, R 291 der Stadtbibliothek,* Part I: Text (Dresden: Marschner, 1908) 182–185; for an analysis of the work see Melitta Weiss-Amer, "Food and Drink in Medical-Dietetic *Fachliteratur* from 1050 to 1400," diss. Toronto, 1989, 126–135.

64. Wolfgang Hirth, "Die Diätetik im Kochbuch des Küchenmeisters Eberhart von Landshut und eine deutsche Regel der Gesundheit nach Arnald von Villanova," *Ostbairische Grenzmarken* 81 (1966): 273–281; and Peter Strauss, "Arnald von Villanova deutsch unter besonderer Berücksichtigung der 'Regel der Gesundheit,'" diss. Heidelberg, 1963.

65. See Christa Hagenmeyer, "Die 'Ordnung der Gesundheit' für Rudolf von Hohenberg: Untersuchungen zur diätetischen Fachprosa des Spätmittelalters mit kritischer Textausgabe," diss. Stuttgart, 1972, 102–219; Hagenmeyer is currently preparing an edition of Konrad's regimen; a transcription of Konrad's dietetic list of foodstuffs is included in Weiss-Amer, "Food and Drink," 296–317; for information on Konrad von Eichstätt, see Günter Kallinich and Karin Figala, "Konrad von Eichstätt, eine Arztpersönlichkeit des Deutschen Mittelalters," *Sudhoffs Archiv* 52 (1969): 341–346.

66. See esp. Hagenmeyer, "Die 'Ordnung der Gesundheit,'" 102–126.

67. Feyl, "Das Kochbuch Meister Eberhards," 12–32; Weiss–Amer, "Die 'Physica' Hildegards von Bingen," 94, esp. n. 23.

68. Hirth, "Studien zu den Gesundheitslehren," 28f.

69. Hirth, 29–31, n. 12; and Schneider, *Deutsche mittelalterliche Handschriften*, 234–237, who describes the treatises on fols. 2r–58v as follows: 2r Rezepte und Notae; 2r–v Jahreszeitenlehre, Auszug aus 'Secretum Secretorum' dt.; 2v–3r Medizinische Aufzeichnungen; 3r–4v

Monatsregimen; 4v–32v Rezeptsammlung, dt. und lat.; 33r–34v Medizinische Wasser; 34v Sechs Heilpflanzen, lat. und dt.; 35r–36v Medizinische Rezepte gegen den Stein; 36v–37v Branntweintraktat; 37v Heilkraft des grünen Kalmus; 38r–47v Exzerpte aus dem Arzneibuch des Ortolfs von Baierland; 48r–55v Heilpflanzen, dt. und lat.; 56r–58v Exzerpte aus den ps.-aristotelischen Problemata physica, lat.

70. Compare the verses "Feniculus verbena rosa celidonia ruta / Ex hys fit aqua que lumina reddit acuta" (fol. 7v) with "Foeniculus, verbena, rosa, chelidonia, ruta: / Ex istis fit aqua quae lumina reddit acuta" in Rolf Schott, *Die Kunst sich gesund zu erhalten: Regimen Sanitatis Salernitanum* (Zurich/Stuttgart: Artemis, 1964) 29.

71. See Gundolf Keil, "Circa instans" in *Verfasserlexikon*, 2nd ed., vol. 1, cols. 1282–1285.

72. See Wolfgang Hirth, "Korpus der Klostermedizin" in *Verfasserlexikon*, 2nd ed., vol. 5, cols. 322–325.

73. Hirth, "Studien zu den Gesundheitslehren," 36–43.

74. Hirth, 38; Eva Hepp, "Die Fachsprache der mittelalterlichen Köche: Ein Lexikon," in Hans Wiswe, *Kulturgeschichte der Kochkunst: Kochbücher und Rezepte aus zwei Jahrtausenden* (Munich: Moos, 1970) 189, "Agraz."

75. The two culinary recipes (fol. 2r) are edited in Feyl, "Das Kochbuch Meister Eberhards," 6f.; the second one is almost identical with recipe 2 (fol. 59r) of the *Eberhard*-cookbook, see Feyl, 85.

76. Schneider, *Deutsche mittelalterliche Handschriften*, 235f.

77. They correspond with all or part of PL I 95, 66, 67, III 43, I 89, 163, III 15, 4, 31, 29, 32, I 42, 36, III 24, I 166.

78. The compiler makes no attempt, e.g., to translate the Salernitan verses from Latin into German rhymed couplets.

79. Gundolf Keil informed me of the sources in a letter, dated June 4, 1992; a detailed analysis of all the sources is included in Barbara Fehringer's dissertation.

80. Barbara Fehringer's preliminary transcription of "Abrothanum-Allium."

81. Gundolf Keil compared the two mansucripts and informed me of his findings in the letter of June 4, 1992.

82. Carl Jessen discovered the Wolfenbüttel and Berlin manuscripts of the *Physica*, as well as the Copenhagen manuscript of the *Causae et Curae*; see Jessen, "Über Ausgaben und Handschriften," esp. 98–104, 111; by 1927, the Brussels manuscript of the *Physica* was also known; see Fischer, *Die Heilige Hildegard von Bingen*, 28.

83. "Die Aufnahme von Hildegard-Traktaten in einen medizinisch-naturkundlichen Sammelband könnte für die Hildegardforschung ein Anstoß sein, auch der natur- und heilkundlichen Handschriftengattung ihre Aufmerksamkeit zuzuwenden. Die spärliche handschriftliche Überlieferung des LSu [Liber subtilitatum diversarum naturarum creaturarum] legt den Gedanken nahe, daß in ma. medizinischen Hss., die weithin unerforscht sind, Hildegard-Material zu entdecken wäre." See Schrader und Führkötter, *Die Echtheit des Schrifttums*, 56.

# Medicine in the *Twelve Books on Rural Practices* of Petrus de Crescentiis*

*William C. Crossgrove*

## 1. Background

It should be noted at the beginning of this chapter that my interest in the *Twelve Books on Rural Practices* derives from work with its late medieval translations into German.[1] There appeared to be a large amount of medical lore in what purports to be a handbook for estate managers, so I decided to examine more closely the role of medicine in the text as it was prepared early in the fourteenth century by the Bolognese lawyer, Peter of Crescent, and transmitted for more than a century and a half in manuscripts before the earliest printed edition. A bit of background is perhaps useful, since this work is not primarily a medical text and thus not normally discussed as part of medical literature.

### *1.1 The Author*

Petrus de Crescentiis, Pietro or Pier de' Crescenzi, or Peter of Crescent was born around 1233 near Bologna (the date is based partly on earlier scholarly traditions and partly on extrapolation backwards from his later career: ca. 1230 is also often given). As a young man he studied medicine and natural science at the University of Bologna, but eventually he turned to law to prepare himself for a professionally remunerative career. He subsequently worked as a lawyer and negotiator for various northern Italian cities, absenting himself from Bologna for many years because of the civil strife that had embroiled his family and forced him to leave his home city in 1274. After relative calm had been restored in Bologna and Peter was nearly 70, he retired and settled on his nearby estate in 1299. Then, encouraged by his friend, the Dominican friar Aimerico Giliani of Piacenza, he returned to a plan he had long nurtured to write a comprehensive guide to estate management based on the best ancient and modern authors, on practices he had observed while traveling through Italy, and on his own experience as a farmer. The work itself was dedicated to King Charles II of Anjou and Jerusalem who died in 1309, and Peter sent it to his friend Aimerico, now the Governor-General of the Dominican Order, for his critical comments. Since Aimerico assumed that position in 1304, scholars have dated the completion of the work to sometime between 1304 and 1309. Peter himself, nearly 90 years old, died in 1320 or early 1321.[2]

## *1.2 The Text*

The text that Peter produced covers a wide range of topics appropriate to managing an estate in Northern Italy, but with references also to other topographical and meteorological conditions. Book One covers matters such as selection of an appropriate site and construction of buildings. The second book is generally about agronomy, horticulture, and techniques of propagation of plants. Book Three discusses field crops. Book Four covers vineyards, vines, and wine making. Book Five concerns itself with trees, and Book Six treats herbs, both domesticated and wild. The short seventh book is divided into two parts, the first on maintaining pastures, and the second on forestry practices. Book Eight describes the construction of pleasure gardens, while Book Nine deals with animal husbandry, fishponds, poultry raising, dovecotes, and beekeeping. Book Ten is devoted to hunting, trapping, and fishing. In Book Eleven the first ten books are briefly summarized, presumably to make it easier for a user to find the appropriate sections for detailed discussion, and the final book is arranged by months with instructions for what should be done in each month to keep an estate running properly. Books Three, Five, and Six are arranged alphabetically according to the name of the plant or tree being discussed, while the other books present their respective subjects in sequences determined by the subject matter itself, or at least by traditional arrangements of that subject matter.

## *1.3 Sources*

Peter relied heavily on his sources, especially Palladius, Varro, Dioscorides, and Pliny among the ancients, while Avicenna and Albertus Magnus are the most frequently cited recent contemporaries. Altogether over forty sources are cited, though quite a few of these were probably taken over from the sources used by Peter rather than coming from the original texts of the authors in question.[3] Some longer sections were copied nearly verbatim, causing the charge of plagiarism to be leveled against the author by various later writers, but many details also appear to have been based on Peter's synthesis of sources or on his own experiences as a farmer.[4]

## *1.4 Manuscripts and Editions*

There has never been a critical edition of Peter's handbook. It was first printed at Augsburg in 1471, and there were five more editions before 1500. It was translated into Italian by the middle of the fourteenth century, into French and German in the fifteenth, Polish in the sixteenth, and Russian in the seventeenth century. There are well over 100 manuscripts of the Latin text extant from the fourteenth through the sixteenth century. The French illuminated manuscripts of the fifteenth century, and woodcuts in many of the early printed editions both of vernacular translations and of the Latin text no doubt contributed to its popularity in the late Middle Ages and early modern times.[5] Will Richter, who published a study of the manuscripts in preparation for an edition that he did not complete before his death, was able to compare twenty-one witnesses from the fourteenth century.[6] Since there is no modern critical edition from which to cite, the 1471 Augsburg *editio princeps* by Johann Schüssler (A), a copy of which is in the Annmary Brown Memorial collection at Brown University and in many other incunable collections, is largely followed here. This printing has no folio or quire numbers, so it is cited by book and chapter. This principle of organization is shared in some fashion by all of the manuscripts I have seen. The text has been corrected with readings from two of the fourteenth century manuscripts representing different branches of Richter's stemma to ensure that we obtain a reasonably accurate picture of the text as it existed in early manuscripts: M = Munich, Bayerische Staatsbibliothek, Cod. lat. 14343; and U = Utrecht, Bibliotheek van de Rijksuniversiteit, Cod. lat. 712. Spelling variations, minor grammatical variants, and changes in word order are generally not noted.

## 2. Medical Content

An overview of the kinds of medical information contained in Peter's handbook provides a convenient starting point. I should emphasize that I am not claiming that medicine plays a prominent role in Peter's text as opposed to its role in other medieval treatises on agriculture. The fact is that Peter's handbook was nearly unique in Italy, France, and Germany for several centuries. Arabic agricultural texts from Spain were translated into Castilian before Peter's time, but they appear to have been little known outside of Iberia,[7] while the French *Hosbandrie* of about 1250 by the Englishman Walter of Henley was known to some extent in France but mainly in French, Latin, and English versions in England.[8] Peter's text competed most directly with the Roman agricultural authorities from whom he drew much of his information, the *Scriptores rei rusticae,* as they were collectively known in early printed editions.[9] These editions usually included the agricultural treatises by Cato,

Varro, Columella, and Palladius, and were among the texts most frequently cited by Peter, but they were not the sources he normally cited on medical matters. For these he referred directly to medical authorities, especially Pliny, Dioscorides, and Gargilius Martialis on herbs, and Avicenna and Albertus Magnus on more theoretical matters. My purpose is not, however, to focus on the specific sources, but rather to examine the medical precepts contained in Peter's handbook and to try to make some sense out of what is included and why.

## *2.1 Preventive Medicine*

Peter begins his first book by noting that the major considerations affecting the choice of an estate are purity of the air, strength of the winds, quality of the water, lie of the land, and its fruitfulness, the latter being reserved as a major topic for the second book.

> 1.1 Qvoniam cultus ruris propter continuos eius labores praecipue fortitudinem habitantium querit. idcirco conueniens michi visum est in hoc primo libro doctrinam tradere de his quae ad cogniconnem salutis locorum habitabilium spectant. et de quibusdam habitaconi necessariis. Nam corpora hominum quibuscumque comodis pecuniarijs debent praeferri. Dicam itaque in primis de cognicone bonitatis loci habitabilis in communi quae quidem attenditur circa quinque. videlicet penes aeris puritatem. ventorum impetuositatem. aquae salubritatem. situs qualitatem. et terre fecunditatem. quorum quattuor in hoc primo libro tractantur. quintum vero traditur in secundo. quae omnia diligenter consideranda sunt. antequem in emptionem praediorum ac fabricam domorum pecunia collata. velox postmodum cum personarum detrimento aut rei familiaris damno. poenitentia non sperata sequatur.
>
> cont. eius labores] cont. labores *U*; querit] requirit *A*; habitantium] habitatorum *M*; pecunia collata] pecuniam collectam *U*.
>
> [Because the cultivation of the land, as a result of the continuous work involved in it, especially requires

> strength of the inhabitants, therefore it seemed appropriate to me in this first book to pass on the teaching of these things which consider the recognition of the health of habitable places, and about such things as are necessary for habitation. For the bodies of people ought to be given preference over any kind of monetary gain. I would thus speak in the first parts about the recognition of the suitability of a habitable place in general which indeed is encompassed in around five points, namely with the purity of air, strength of winds, wholesomeness of water, the quality of the site, and the fecundity of the earth, of which four are treated in this first book, and the fifth is discussed in the second. The points are all to be considered in detail before money is collected for purchase of lands and construction of buildings, or quickly thereafter unhoped for punishment with harm of persons and diminution of family fortunes can follow.]

The next four chapters of Book One treat the first four topics in terms of their effects on health, with Avicenna being cited in each instance. The final eight chapters, drawing especially on Palladius, go into details of providing a secure site, laying out a courtyard, digging a well, constructing buildings, hiring a manager, if appropriate, and laying in supplies. The opening chapters on air, winds, water, and location draw partly on Roman agricultural texts, but they also place us in the context of "Regimen sanitatis" literature, with notions ultimately going back to Hippocrates that maintenance of health is the best way to fight disease.

The theme of preventive medicine is again picked up in Book Eight, on pleasure gardens. The reason for having such an artificially constructed garden is that it provides the soul with pleasure and thereby preserves the health of the body, for the humors of the body are at all times dependent on the soul.

> 8. Incipit liber octauus de viridarijs et rebus delectabilibus ex arboribus herbis et fructu ipsorum artificialiter agendis.
>
> In superioribus libris tractatum est de arboribus et herbis secumdum quod vtilia corpori humano existunt. Nunc vero de eisdem dicendum est secundum quod anime rationali delectationem afferunt. et consequenter corporis salutem conseruant. quia complexio corporis animi semper adheret affectui.

delectationem] delecta communes *A*.

[Here Book Eight begins on pleasure gardens and delightful things achieved by skillful management from trees, herbs and the fruit of them.

In the previous books trees and herbs have been discussed according to how advantages accrue to the human body. Now indeed things must be discussed in terms of how they provide pleasure to the reasoning soul and consequently preserve the health of the body, since the condition of the body always corresponds to the disposition of the spirit.]

Especially large and elaborate gardens are appropriate for kings to the extent that they earn the right to greater forms of relaxation by virtue of their deeds:

8.3 . . . in tali itaque viridario non semper delectetur rex. sed aliquando cum serijs necessarijsque satisfecerit rebus renouetur in eo. glorificans deum excelsum. qui omnium bonarum et licitarum delectaconem principium est et causa.

bonarum . . . delectaconem] bonorum delectaconumque auctor *A*.

[. . . a king should, however, not always be delighted by such a garden, but should only occasionally be renewed in it when he has fulfilled his duty with serious and necessary things glorifying God the highest, who is the origin and cause of all good and licit pleasures.]

Parts of the book on pleasure gardens are taken verbatim from Albertus Magnus, as we have noted earlier in quoting Fischer. It is not inconceivable that Peter, who was only about thirty years younger than Albert, could even have encountered the famous Dominican during the latter's many stays in Italy, but Albert, who died in 1280, spent most of his later years north of the Alps. Peter's long-standing relationship with the Dominican order is reflected both in some documentary evidence that he did legal work for Dominican friars and in his singling out of his friend Aimerico, the Governor-General of the Dominicans, to read and comment on his text.[10] The specific physiological claim, that psychic balance contributes to the humoral balance of the body, fits in well with the notions underlying "regimen" literature. Peter's use of this precept to justify the creation of a pleasure garden seems to resonate both with Classical notions of relaxation from the cares of the day and with the practice of reserving parts of monastic gardens for contemplation.

## *2.2 Materia Medica*

Books Three (on field crops), Five (on trees), and Six (on herbs) share some common features. All three are organized alphabetically, as I noted earlier; all three discuss types of plants, and share certain common features in the structure of the individual chapters. The typical chapter begins with (a) the name of the plant; (b) details on appropriate soil, cultivation, planting, propagation, or finding in the wild, depending on the plant; (c) uses of the plant for food, fiber, or building; and (d) medicinal uses of the plant. One or more of these features is often missing, but a significant number of the chapters contain the full panoply. In most cases the medicinal uses are introduced by identifying the qualities and degrees of the plant in terms of the system of humoral pathology. Millet, for example, is said to be cold in the first degree and dry in the second; according to Isaac:

> Book 3 [De milio]. . . . Milium secundum ysaac frigidum est in primo gradu. siccum in secundo. testatur hoc leuitas et concauitas eius et viscositas et ventositatisque absentia. minus nutrit ceteris granis ex quibus fit panis. gratia tamen sue siccitatis confortatiuum est stomachi et aliorum membrorum corporis. Diureticum est. et ideo assatur ad ignem. et ad torconem doloremque ventris calidum superponitur. Causa autem sue siccitatis et nutrimenti nimium non est accipiendum ab his qui carnes suas augmentari et impinguari desiderant. nec ab eis qui in corporibus suis laudabilem sanguinem generari volunt. sed ab illis tamen a quibus refrigeratio aut confortatio humorumque superfluorum desiccatio appetitur.
>
> secundo] secundo gradu *A*; absencia] habundantia *A*; tamen sue] tamen *A*; ideo] idem *A*; torconem] corrosionem *A*; Causa autem] Causa *A*; in corporibus suis] in corpor-

ibus *A*; volunt] desiderant *M*; sed ab illis] sed *A*; humorumque] humorum *A*.

[[On millet]. . . . Millet according to Isaac is cold in the first degree and dry in the second. Its lightness and hollowness and stickiness and absence of gas demonstrates this. It is less nutritious than other grain from which one makes bread. But by virtue of its dryness it is a relaxant to the stomach and to all other organs of the body. It is a diuretic and therefore it is roasted on a fire and applied hot for churning and pain of the belly. But because of its dryness and insufficience of nutrition it is not acceptable for those who wish to augment their flesh and get fatter, nor for those who want to generate good blood in their bodies, but on the other hand it is sought by the ones for whom cooling or comforting and the drying of superfluous humors is desired.]

Occasionally the more elaborate system familiar from the *Circa instans* is evident, as when Peter notes that garlic (*Alleum*) is warm and dry in the middle of the fourth degree. Peter presumably derives his information from various sources and he is aware that they do not always agree. For the barberry bush, discussed as one of the trees in Book Five, he notes that it is cold and dry in the second degree, but in the third, according to Avicenna:

Book 5 [De berberis]. Berberi est fructus cuiusdam arboris parue valde spinose. similis arbori maligranati. et sunt rotundi tales ut fructus spine albe aliquantulum oblongi quasi subnigri. plantantur ut malapunica. frigidi sunt et sicci in secundo gradu. valent contra febrilem discrasiam. sirupus ex eis et zuccaro factus. contra calefactionem epatis. puluis eorum cum succo solatri conficiatur. et superponatur epati. Auicenna dicit quod sint frigidi et sicci in tercio gradu. dicit etiam et sunt vincentes coleram et scindunt sitim valde huismodi fructus. arbustula optima est pro clausuris et sepibus si haberetur plantarum copia. que quidem per sationem fructus vel seminarij eius facile haberi potest.

*This chapter (and all of Books Four and Five) is missing in M*; similis arbori maligranati] sicut arbor maligranate *U*;

rotundi tales] rotundi rubei quasi nigri *A*; scindunt] abscindunt *U*; seminarij] seminis eius *A*.

[[On barberry]. Barberry is the fruit of a certain shrub that is very thorny, similar to the pomegranate tree, and they are round like the fruits of the hawthorn, a bit oblong and somewhat blackish. They are planted like pomegranates. They are cold and dry in the second degree. They are effective against febrile distress. A syrup is made from them with sugar against overheating of the liver. A powder of them is prepared with the juice of nightshade and placed over the liver. Avicenna says that they are cold and dry in the third degree. And furthermore he says they can overcome choler, and the fruits in this way greatly quench thirst. A planting of them is excellent for enclosures and hedges if an abundance of plants was established which indeed is easily possible to have by a sowing of the fruit or with a nursery.]

The point to be noted is that Peter presumably drew on both agricultural writers and medical authorities for his information on plants. If the plant grew mainly in the wild rather than being cultivated, the medical uses were likely to be the predominant theme, as in the case of burning bush.

Book 6 [De dyptamo]. Dyptamus qui alio nomine dicitur fraxinella quia frondes habet ad modum fraxini calida. et sicca. est in iiij° gradu. radix est cuiusdam herbe simili nomine appellate. quae in locis calidis lapidosis et siccis praecipue reperitur. habet autem ipsa radix virtutem attrahendi consumendi et dissoluendi venenum. Contra morsum venenatorum animalium ipsa herba valet radix trita superponatur. Succus etiam eius cum vino detur. puluis eius cum succo mente conficiatur et superponatur et potui detur. Isidorus insuper dicit quod est tante virtutis ut ferrum a corpore extrahat vnde eius pabulo fere percusse eijciunt sagittas corpori infixas.

iiij°] tercio *A*; radix] radix eius *A*; autem ipsa] autem praecipue ipsa *A*; venenatorum] venatorum *A*; vnde] vnde et *A*.

[[On burning bush]. Burning bush, which is called little ash by another name because it has leaves similar to the ash, is hot and dry in the fourth degree. Its root is called

> by a similar name of a certain herb which is found principally in stony places that are warm and dry. Furthermore, this root has the power of drawing, consuming and dissolving poison. Against the bite of venomous animals this herb helps if the ground up root is applied. And the juice of it should be given with wine. Its powder is prepared with mint juice and given to be drunk. Isidore says above that it is of such strength that it draws iron out from a body so that by eating it wounded animals usually eject arrows stuck in their body.]

## *2.3 Wine and Vinegar as Medicinals*

The third type of medical information is contained in the final chapters of Book Four on vineyards. The bulk of this book, which draws heavily on Greek *Geoponika* chapters translated by Burgundio of Pisa in the twelfth century, is devoted to the selection, propagation, and pruning of vines, the harvesting and processing of grapes, and the storing, handling, and manipulation of wine. It is also noted already in the first chapter that one of the main uses of the grape is in preparing medicines because of its cooling and antiseptic properties. Chapter 19 discusses the virtues of grapes and notes that the three parts—pits, juice, and skins—have different medicinal properties, and that these properties vary with the ripeness of the grapes. The next twenty-four chapters deal with the grape harvest, processing into wine, storing and tapping wine barrels, and manipulations to flavor the wine or disguise bad wine. Chapter 44 describes how to make vinegar, and the following chapter goes into its various medicinal uses, including the preparation of simple or flavored oximel—two parts vinegar and one part honey—one of the major bases for medical syrups. The following chapter, one of the longest in Peter's entire text, discusses the medicinal uses of wine in considerable detail, classifying different wines by age, color, and taste, and concluding with a warning against drunkenness. These last two chapters of Book Four have the form of genuine medical treatises, the kinds of texts frequently compiled together in medical handbooks.

Avicenna is cited once in the vinegar text, with Isaac cited once and Galen twice in the wine text.

## *2.4 Veterinary Medicine*

Book Nine, dealing with animal husbandry, includes significant amounts of material on veterinary medicine. The relative importance of horses in medieval Europe is reflected in the fact that 57 of the 105 chapters of Book Nine deal with horses, and 48 of these 57 chapters are concerned with treating their diseases and injuries. Chapter 38, on treating "spinella" with cauterization, is a typical example:

> 9.38 De spinellis et cura eius.
> Hic morbus qui spinella vocatur fit subtus garectum in iunctura ossis. eiusdem garecti in vtroque latere. et quandoque in vno tantum. creans super os ad magnitudinem auellane. vel magis reprimens iuncturam in tantum. quod equus multotiens cogitur claudicare. et accidit equo his causis ut turba. cura. dicte spinelle sunt decente coquende atque curande ut praedicte cocture in omnibus curantur.
>
> quandoque] aliquando *M*; curande] curande dilgente *A*.
>
> [On spinella and its cure.
> The disease called spinella occurs beneath the hock in the joint of the bone on both sides of the hock, and sometimes so much on one that it grows over the bone to the size of a hazelnut or more, hindering the joint so much that the horse frequently is driven to limp and it happens to the horse for these reasons as a disturbance. Treatment: the aforementioned spinellas are appropriate for cauterizing and curing just as the previously mentioned things are cured by cauterization in all instances.]

For most of the other creatures mentioned, including cattle, sheep, goats, dogs, chickens, and bees, there are some references to treatment of illnesses or injuries, but nothing as detailed as in the case of horses. This fairly accurately reflects the amount of material transmitted in medieval texts on veterinary medicine, including that of Jordanus Ruffus, perhaps the best known medieval Latin tract.[11] Only horses are usually the subject of independent tracts, while treatment of other farm animals is typically mentioned only in occasional recipes or as accretions to books on treating horses.

## 3. Medicine in an Agricultural Handbook

Having provided an overview of the medical content in Peter's book, I would like now to turn in more detail to the question of what these medical precepts are doing in an agricultural handbook. The material will be discussed in reverse order, beginning with veterinary medicine.

### *3.1 Veterinary Medicine*

The only people who somewhat approximated modern veterinarians in medieval Europe appear to have been the marshalls in charge of the stables of great lords. Ordinary farmers, from peasants to estate managers, presumably had to provide their own veterinary medicine on most occasions. The result was, as I noted before, that only the treatment of horses became the subject of an extensive written literature, while the treatment of other animals was largely a matter of transmitted practice. Something of this is reflected in Peter's discussion of sheep. With nine chapters, sheep raising is the third most detailed treatment in Book Nine, trailing only the fifty-seven chapters devoted to horses and the twelve chapters on beekeeping. Much of the detail is devoted to selecting, breeding, and shearing sheep, as well as making cheese from sheep's milk. There is also a short chapter on the diseases of sheep, but after a few perfunctory observations, Peter notes that other diseases are likely to affect sheep, too, but the herders who spend all their time with the animals are supposed to know how to deal with these problems:

> 9.73 De morbo ouium et cura eius.
> Nascitur eis gossum sub gula. ex fluxu humorum a capite descendentium. ac perforatur ibi pellis. et inde quasi aquae paulatim egreditur. et curantur. Item paciuntur

grossiciem splenis. et inflantur. et hoc sepius de mense maij et aprilis ex multitudine sanguinis grossi et viscosi. ex quo sepe subito moriuntur. ac confert eis vnum stetum duorum digitorum. ponere intus nares. et facere quod multus egrediatur sanguis. ex quo quaedam liberantur. et quaedam nichilominus moriuntur. Item paciuntur febres quae cognosci et curari possunt ut dictum est. de febribus in tractatu boum. possunt etiam eis alie accidere egritudines. quas cognoscere et curare pastores nouerent expertissimi. qui totis temporibus in sola custodia ouium exercentur et in talibus solummodo student.

sepius] sepe *A*; ex quo sepe] ex hoc sepe *M*; ponere] ponetur *A*; multus] multum *A*; ex quo quaedam] quaedam *M*; totis temporibus suis] eorum temporum *A*; et in] in *A*.

[On disease of sheep and the cure of it.
A growth arises in them beneath the gullet from the movement of humors descending from the head, and the hide is perforated there, and from there a watery substance slowly is forced out and they are cured. Likewise they suffer enlargement of the spleen and are bloated, and this is more often in the month of May or April from the multitude of coarse and viscous blood from which they often suddenly die, and one takes for them a stick of two fingers' size to put inside the nostrils and to cause a lot of blood to flow out. Some are freed from that and some die nonetheless. Likewise they suffer from fevers which can be recognized and cured as has been said about fevers in the treatise on cattle. Moreover other sicknesses can also happen to them, which the most expert shepherds were supposed to know how to recognize and treat, who occupy all of their time only with the custody of the sheep and pay attention solely to such things.]

Thus not only is veterinary medicine an overall responsibility of the estate manager, but the responsibility for particular animals devolves onto those directly in charge of caring for them, and they are presumably supposed to have learned proper techniques of treatment as part of their practical training.

## *3.2 Plant Pathology*

Medicine indirectly also provides a kind of model for plant pathology, not something that was normally recognized as an independent branch of knowledge. The first five chapters of Book Two provide a general theory of plant growth, followed by sixteen chapters on grafting and plant propagation, fertilization, tilling, planting times, and selection of good soil, while the last two chapters discuss construction of hedges and dikes. In the opening chapters, Peter cites Albertus on the seven factors conditioning plant growth, and Aristotle on the comparison of plants to animals, with the earth being like a uterus, the moisture like blood in animals, and fibers analogous to veins and tendons. This analogical thinking conditions a few recommendations for treating plants. Thus, boring a hole near the roots is supposed to relieve overheating that leads to the production of excessive foliage and rotting fruit, and the analogy is with bloodletting:

> 2.4 De diuisione plantarum per suas partes integrales.
> . . . Sunt plante voraces dicte et abstinentes. propter suarum radicum disposicones contrarias. raras enim et porosas et calidas habentes radices multum trahunt de nutrimento plus autem quam converti possit et terminari a natura arboris. et tunc arbor generabit fructus vermiculos et putrescentes si non exsudet. vel aliter emittat superfluum humidum. in iuuentute autem plantarum hoc maxime accidit propter calorem iuuentutis earum. Aliquando autem curantur ex hoc quod perforantur iuxta radicem. ibi enim exit superfluum humidum sicut per fleubothomiam. . . .
>
> abstinentes] abstinentes dicte et *A*; plus autem] plus *A*.
>
> [On the division of plants according to their essential parts.
> . . . There are plants called voracious and abstemious according to the contrasting dispositions of their roots. For those having loose and porous and hot roots draw a lot from the nourishment, more even than can be digested and be limited by the nature of the tree. And then the tree produces wormy and rotting fruit if it does not sweat or otherwise eliminate the excess moisture. Moreover this occurs mostly during the youth of plants in keeping with

> the heat of their youth. But sometimes they are cured by this that they are perforated next to the root where then the excess liquid exits as if in bloodletting.]

Measures such as these are unlikely to have done much more than allow easier access for plant parasites or insects, but the point I want to make is that animal medicine seemingly provided a possible model for plant pathology to medieval authors. Some measures recommended to restore the health of a dying tree, for instance, may have been effective, but it was almost certainly not because practitioners had an appropriate model for plant diseases.

The treatment of vines was relatively advanced, presumably representing their importance as a cash crop. Chapter 17 of Book Four specifically addresses damaged and diseased vines and treatments for them. Weeds should be removed; shade and mulch can prevent damage from excess sun; rodent damage can be prevented by poison, by planting thorn bushes around vineyards, or by digging and fencing around the vines; frost damage can be minimized by proper pruning or mulching or by use of late varieties; insects should be removed and squashed, a job reserved for a bug brigade of women and children; mildew can be prevented by using resistant grape varieties; vines damaged by hoes can be bound up; people and dogs should be kept away; varieties that do not taste good but make good wine should be planted along exposed areas to keep passersby from picking the grapes; noisemakers should be used against starlings; and finally, against storms you should pray to God. All in all, this is a fairly comprehensive and effective set of measures, but one based on the experience of vintners rather than on effective precepts about plant pathology.

### *3.3 Human Medicine*

As for the human medicine in Peter's handbook, one can probably assume that he was generally conversant with prevailing medical theories both as a result of his early studies in Bologna as a young man and because of his extensive reading and contacts with intellectuals during his professional life. It is not surprising, then, that he should adopt widely accepted notions concerning the non-naturals, namely the role of air and water in selection of a healthy farm site and emotional balance as a justification for a pleasure garden. His sources provided him with ample precedent, and it seems likely that Peter was receptive to this view. Security from disease and security from ill-meaning people actually seem to go together in a belief that people are individually responsible for their well-being. Chapter 6 of Book One notes, for instance, that it is not good to build too close to ponds and marshy areas because little creatures (called *minuta animalia* and *bestiolae*) grow in them that can enter people or animals through their noses or mouths and cause disease.

> 1.5 De situ loci habitabilis et de cognicone bonitatis et malicie sue.
> . . . Aduertendum est si aquae erunt loca palustria et propter easdem causas. et quia cum arescant crescunt animalia quaedam minuta quae non possunt oculi consequi. et per aera intus in corpus per os et nares perueniunt. et efficiunt difficiles morbos. Item scropha. vitandum est inquit ne in eam partem spectet villa ex quae ventus grauior afflare solet. neue in conualle caua sed pocius in sublimi loco edifices. eo quod cum perflatur. si quod est quod aduersarium inferatur facilius discutitur. preterea locus qui a sole tota die illustratus salubrior est. quia ac bestiole si quae perpetue nascuntur et inferuntur aut efflantur aut aritudine cito pereunt.
>
> Aduertendum] Animaduertendum *A*; quia cum] quia *M*; est inquit] inquid *U*; vitandum . . . quae] vitandum quam *M*; neue] ne *A*; est quod] est ibi *A*; preterea] propterea *A*; aut efflantur] aut nimbi efflantur *M*; aut afflantur *A*.
>
> [On the site of a habitable place and the recognition of its goodness and badness.
> . . . It is to be noted if there are waters and marshy places and for the same reasons, namely because when they dry up certain tiny creatures grow which cannot be followed by the eye and which get into the body through the air via the mouth and the nostrils and produce serious diseases. Likewise Scropha: it is to be avoided, he says, to give thought to that place for a villa either from which the wind is apt to blow more strongly or to hollow valleys, but rather you should build in a high place, in one where it can be blown through, for if it happens that one is

> attacked, it is easier for an enemy to be driven away. What is more, a place which is lit up all day by the sun is more healthy because the little creatures constantly being born and carried in either are blown out or perish quickly from the dryness.]

For the same reason it is good to have ample sunshine entering houses because it kills the beasties that get into the house or blow in on the wind. A high place not only avoids the strong winds of valleys, but also has the further advantage of being more secure against robbers and thieves. Thus, the preventive measures seem like a natural part both of Peter's intellectual background and of agricultural literature.

The medical recipes incorporated into the chapters on plants and the treatises on medicinal uses of vinegar and wine are less obvious parts of an agricultural treatise. Such material is not systematically prefigured in the Roman agricultural literature. Medicine is not entirely lacking, as perhaps best reflected in the lengthy discourse on the virtues of cabbage in Cato's *De Agri Cultura*, a text from the first half of the second century B.C., claimed by some to be the earliest extant Roman prose text and a source cited fifteen times by Peter. But none of the Roman agricultural texts approach Peter's either in the variety of plants discussed or in the amount of information on medical properties. Pliny and Dioscorides, the latter presumably available in a Latin translation, are each cited more than twenty times, mainly as medical authorities in the sections on plants. Peter himself provides us with the reason for the inclusion of this material. In the introduction to Book Six, he says that he intends to include in his alphabetically arranged discussion of garden plants those plants that grow in the wild without the help of human intervention, because many of these plants are especially useful in the treatment and prevention of diseases. Knowledge of such things is useful to all people and especially to country dwellers, where composite medicines are not readily available. Put differently, the well-prepared estate manager must himself know how to provide medical care because it is quite likely that it will not be available to him from a qualified physician:

> Book 6. Incipit liber sextus de ortis et de natura et vtilitate tam herbarum que seruntur in eis quaeque ceterarum quae in alijs locis sine hominum industria naturaliter nascuntur.
>
> Tractaturus de ortis et de industria cultus ipsorum et de omnibus herbis quae propter alimentum humani corporis seruntur in eis dicam de his mixtim. secundum ordinem alphabeti. que sine hominis ministerio ex ipsa elementorum commixtione in alijs nascuntur locis. quibus frequenter vtimur. ut earum virtute corpora in aliquae egritudine lapsa ad salutem pristinam reducantur. vel ante lapsum sana seruentur. huiusmodi namque cognitio valde vtilis erit omnibus et praecipue habitantibus rura vbi medicinarum compositarum copia non habetur.
>
> sextus] quattuor *M (since Books 4 and 5 are lacking)*; nascuntur] nascustur *M*; humani corporis] humanum corporum *M*; in eis] etiam *M*; ipsa] ipsorum *A*; huiusmodi] huius *U*.
>
> [Here begins the sixth book on gardens and the nature and use both of herbs which are sown in them and those others which arise naturally in other places without the intervention of people.
> Setting out to treat gardens and the effort of cultivation of them and of all herbs which are sown in them as food for the human body, I would speak following alphabetical order of them together with those which arise without the attention of man from the same mixture of elements in other places from which we make use of them in order from the strength of them to restore bodies fallen into some diseases to pristine health or to keep them healthy before the onset. Truly, knowledge of this kind would be very useful for all and especially for dwellers in the country where an abundance of composite medicines is not available.]

This hardly comes as a stunning insight to us: We have generally been aware that academic medicine did not extend its reach much beyond the larger towns where wealthy patrons could afford to support university-educated physicians. It seems, however, that Peter wants to suggest that if academic physicians are not available, the next best thing is for the educated estate manager to provide treatment using the knowledge that has been accumulated by academic medicine. I would argue that what we have here is a step in the direction of reliance on written sources for medical treatment in the secular world, even when academically trained medical practitioners are not available. Thus the recipes collected in early medieval monasteries in some sense have their parallel in the recipes incorporated into Peter's handbook on agriculture. Both suggest a possible bias against the traditional practitioner in favor of learned medicine, even if that medicine, is to be practiced by a nonspecialist.

## 4. Conclusion

In concluding, I would note that Peter of Crescent's compilation of *Twelve Books on Rural Practices* was popular both in Latin and in vernacular translations from the time it was first composed, but it really came into its own with the early printed editions of both the original and translations, presumably a reflection of the expanding audience of potential readers. Various parts of it were also extracted and transmitted separately, especially the book on hunting, the sections on animal husbandry, and the wine book. Yet none of the medical content has to my knowledge been identified as the source of subsequent medical texts. This is not surprising, since the number of herbals, medical handbooks, rules of health, and treatises on specific aspects of medicine continued to grow throughout the Middle Ages, both in Latin versions and in translations. Anyone wanting to prepare a medical treatise was likely to have access to the same sources Peter used, or to improved versions of them. Furthermore, the later compilers of home handbooks tended to put together a series of independent treatises on each of the subjects they wished to include. Medical treatises certainly played a large role in these compilations. The medical content of Peter's handbook is indeed in some sense its least original part. But it was also an integral part of the kind of agricultural handbook he envisioned producing, and it may have been one of the most heavily used portions of the text for some users who acquired a copy. I have not done a systematic comparison of manuscripts and early editions, but in at least one of the texts that I have examined, the medical sections were liberally annotated with marginalia from users. Peter's view of the practice of medicine on rural estates run by people who were sufficiently literate to read his handbook was probably an accurate reflection of the state of medical belief and practice at the beginning of the fourteenth century and for a few centuries after that.

## NOTES

*My thanks to Michael Gleason of the Department of Comparative Literature at Brown University for offering suggestions for improving my translations of the Latin passages.

1. See "Das landwirtschaftliche Handbuch von *Petrus de Crescentiis* in der deutschen Fassung des *Bruder Franciscus*," *Sudhoffs Archiv* 78 (1994): 97–106.

2. The most comprehensive study of Petrus de Crescentiis was prepared in Bologna in commemoration of his presumed 700th birthday: *Pier de'Crescenzi (1233–1321), Studi e documenti* a cura di Tommaso Alfonsi, Roberto Bozzelli, Ludovico Frati, Alessandro Ghigi, Giovanni Livi, Arturo Palmieri, Napoleone Passerini, Lino Sighinolfi, Albano Sorbelli, Francesco Todaro, Gaspare Ungarelli, Dino Zucchini, and Guido Zucchino (Societa Agraria di Bologna), (Bologna: Licinio Cappelli, 1933). See also the article on Pietro de' Crescenzi by P. Toubert in Volume 30 of the *Dizionario Biografico degli Italiani* (Rome: Instituto della Enciclopedia Italiana, 1984) 649–657.

3. The sources from Antiquity were studied by Anna Röding in her Göteborg dissertation: *Studier till Petrus de Crescentiis och hans antika källor* (Göteborg: Elanders Boktryckeri Aktiebolag, 1927). There has been no comparably detailed study of Petrus's modern (i.e., medieval) sources.

4. Hermann Fischer, e.g., states that Petrus had "glatt abgeschrieben" from Albertus Magnus in his chapter on gardens (*Mittelalterliche Pflanzenkunde,* Geschichte der Wissenschaften, Geschichte der Botanik, vol. 2, [Munich: Verlag der Münchener Drucke, 1929] 171), while Will Richter, on the other hand, calls the *Ruralia commoda* "eines der größten und interessantesten 'wissenschaftlichen' Werke des Abendlandes" (*Mittellateinisches Jahrbuch* 16 [1981]: 225). One possible source not specifically mentioned by Petrus could be Vincent of

Beauvais, given Petrus's close relationship to the Dominican Order, but no one has to my knowledge examined this question.

5. See Robert G. Calkins, "Piero de' Crescenzi and the Medieval Garden" in *Medieval Gardens*, ed. Elizabeth B. MacDougall, Dumbarton Oaks Colloquium on the History of Landscape Architecture 9 (Washington, D.C.: Dumbarton Oaks, 1986) 155–173.

6. "Die Überlieferung der 'Ruralia commoda' des Petrus de Crescentiis im 14. Jahrhundert," *Mittellateinisches Jahrbuch*, 16 (1981): 223–275. When the oral version of this paper was delivered in Kalamazoo, a representative of E. J. Brill Publishers indicated during the discussion that Richter's edition was finished in a handwritten version that Brill would like to publish. Unfortunately, they feel that this cannot be done unless someone first transcribes the German script into a more readable version. This is presumably the same text that was made available to Clemens Alexander Wimmer for his *Geschichte der Gartentheorie* (Darmstadt: Wissenschaftliche Buchgesellschaft, 1989) by Richter's daughter, Dr. Reinhilt Richter-Bergmeier of Hannover. Wimmer prints a section of Petrus's chapter on gardens (pp. 26–29).

7. Cf. G.S. Colin, in B. Lewis, C. Pellat, and J. Schacht, eds., *The Encyclopedia of Islam*, rev. ed. (Leiden: E.J. Brill; London: Luzac & Co., 1965) vol. 2, 901–902.

8. Cf. Dorothea Oschinsky, *Walter of Henley and Other Treatises on Estate Management and Accounting* (Oxford: The Clarendon Press, 1971). I owe this reference to James Marchand in response to an inquiry posted to the electronic discussion group MEDTEXTL.

9. The first edition of the Roman agricultural writers was edited by George Merula and published by Nicolaus Jensen in Venice in 1472. Among the most notable later editions of the *Scriptores rei rusticae* are those of Johann Matthias Gesner (1735) and Johann Gottlieb Schneider (1794–1796).

10. Cf. Tommaso Alfonsi, "Il Padre Aimerico Giliani e Pier de' Crescenzi" in Alfonsi et al. (n. 2), 49–60.

11. The relationship of the "source of veterinary medicine of Albertus Magnus" discussed by Klaus-Dietrich Fischer ("Zur Erstveröffentlichung einer spätmittelenglischen Pferdeheilkunde [aus Ms. Sloane 2584] nebst Beobachtungen zu ihrer lateinischen, von Albertus Magnus benutzten Vorlage" in Gundolf Keil, ed., *Gelêrter der arzenîe, ouch apotêker. Beiträge zur Wissenschaftsgeschichte: Festschrift zum 70. Geburtstag von Willem F. Daems*. Würzburger medizinhistorische Forschungen, 24 [Pattensen/Hannover: Horst Wellm Verlag, 1982] 221–

238) has not to my knowledge been examined as a possible source for material in Petrus's chapters on veterinary medicine.

# Medicine in Medieval Calendar Manuscripts*

*Faith Wallis*

## 1. Computus and Computus Manuscripts

In the medieval period, the science of calculating time and the art of constructing calendars comprised a loosely defined body of knowledge and technique called *computus*.[1] The extent of interest in the calendar and the various problems it posed is reflected in the enormous number of manuscripts that contain computus texts and tables. This essay is a preliminary report on a project to catalogue and study the medical texts and images that appear in computus manuscripts, a project that is, in turn, an outgrowth of a larger enterprise: a general history of, and guide to the computus based on the manuscripts.[2] In order to situate the medical project within its larger context, I will begin by considering briefly what kind of knowledge computus is, and what its manuscript vehicles look like.

As a genre of knowledge, computus bears little resemblance to a modern science or even a medieval *disciplina*. To begin with, it is a branch of learning with no direct ancestor within the ancient canon of the sciences, and no lineal modern descendent. But more important, computus is embodied in and conveyed through forms which are not like those of other sciences. It is not built up from a syllabus of canonized texts; in fact, it is for the most part, and certainly in its most formative period, not built around texts at all, but rather around tables.

Even the major medieval textbook on the subject, Bede's *De temporum ratione* (A.D. 725), is fundamentally an extended commentary on the two basic tables of the computus: the Julian solar calendar (with additional tables or formulae to adapt it to any given year), and the Paschal table, or table showing the dates of Easter and its dependent feasts for a given sequence of years. In the final analysis, the history of computus is the history of the fortunes of these two tables. Hence, it is a science with a strong graphic orientation, and in consequence, it is indissolubly wedded to the manuscripts through which it is conveyed.

Moreover, these two tables attracted into their respective orbits other materials not strictly calendrical in nature, but associated with the calendar by analogy, or for paedagogical reasons. The Julian solar calendar arrived at the threshold of the Middle Ages already encrusted with zodiacal and meteorological information and admonition, to which medieval computists eagerly added.[3] This impulse to festoon the bald list of dates and feasts with astronomical, agricultural, or medical notations also has strong roots in the ancient Roman *menologia rustica*.[4] These monumental calendars did not contain the usual calendrical apparatus found in urban *fasti*, such as nundinal letters (the letters A–H, repeated sequentially throughout the year, standing for an eight-day "week" used primarily to fix market days). Rather, the months were illustrated by their zodiac signs, and the entrance of the Sun into each zodiac sign was always flagged. So were the lengths of the day and the night, the major feasts of the month, and the agricultural tasks to be accomplished. The focus of these *menologia*, in brief, was on the seasonal patterns of the natural world.

This kind of material proved attractive to Christian calendar-makers of the patristic period, because it furnished them with a morally unobjectionable substitute for the overtly pagan feasts of the old civil calendar. When Polemius Silvius was commissioned in A.D. 449 to make a calendar for a Christian bishop, he was faced with the task of trying to disinfect a conventional civil calendar. But stripping off the pagan and imperial festivals would have left him with nothing but a bald list of dates. This would hardly have constituted a calendar in his or his patron's eyes, for in the Roman tradition, a calendar was fundamentally a list of *named* days.[5] But what would he name the days? The number of Christian fixed feasts was still very small, so Polemius elected to fill the embarrassing gaps with meteorological and seasonal indicators, as well as other paraphernalia such as Egyptian Days, already found in the calendar of Filocalus. Inspiration for such a move undoubtedly came from the old Roman tradition of the *menologia rustica*. Further precedents were furnished by Roman elementary educational practice, which compelled youngsters to memorize lists of places, objects, natural phenomena, and so forth, including lists of the months. The persistent influence of the months' list can be detected in the pedantic calendar poetry of Ausonius and other writers of late Antiquity, poetry which in turn was often included amongst the optional additions to the pages of calendars. These calendar poems are of interest to medical historians, for their usual theme was either the weather appropriate to each month, with the consequences of this for agriculture and hygiene, or the Egyptian Days. They are ubiquitous in medieval calendars.[6]

The Paschal table likewise had a tendency to carry a train of extracalendrical addenda. The type of Paschal table that eventually prevailed in the West was based on a nineteen-year lunar cycle perfected in Alexandria, the major centre of computus research in late Antiquity. For many centuries, however, it was in competition with other cycles, so it tended to travel with a baggage of apologetic texts that defended its accuracy and orthodoxy. But as these tables crossed North Africa and Italy in the sixth and seventh centuries, they also took on board additional tables and formulae, as well as useful supplementary materials such as notes on astronomy and mathematics, and even peripheral elements (texts on medicine, music, grammar, and tables of weights and measures) that attached themselves to the computus by a kind of associative attraction.[7] Some of the earliest surviving Western computus manuscripts already contain a halo of noncomputistical materials, some of which can be described as propaedeutic to the computus (e.g., astronomy, cosmology, and mathematics), but much of which is simply analogous to the computus, the common element being time and its measurement. Medicine was one of these analogous subjects, for the prognostic and therapeutic systems of ancient medicine paid close attention to the phases of the Moon, the seasons, and the age of the patient.

This accretive, associative mode of organizing knowledge, so typical of early medieval theology, for example, is a reflection of early medieval styles of education, which stressed practical training for priestly duties or for the monastic life. Such vocational training, in marked contrast to ancient schooling or the university education of the post-twelfth-century period, was not organized into syllabi and curricula, but conveyed through guided reading, precept, example, and informal instruction by a mentor.[8] The calendar was an essential component of this clerical training, and because the construction of the calendar was at least until the eighth century a matter of considerable controversy and experimentation, computus was an enterprise in which there was much research and interest. For these two reasons, the computus manuscript's already pronounced encyclopaedic character was willingly exploited as a sort of filing cabinet for the scattered fragments of ancient scientific erudition found on the pages of Pliny and Isidore, erudition which, by the vocational criteria of early medieval clerical education, would otherwise have been ignored as superfluous *curiositas*.[9] This encyclopaedic tendency is reflected not only in the non-computistical elements in Bede's *De temporum ratione*,[10] but in the shape of countless medieval computus manuscripts. A typical "encyclopaedic" computus manuscript will group one or more of these "halo" topics around a dominant core composed of calendar, Paschal tables, and computus texts and formulae.

The eleventh century is in every way the watershed of the history of medieval computus, and the changes in the discipline are closely bound up with the shift from a vocational to a curricular education. At the beginning of this period, we see monastic and secular schoolmasters like Gerbert and Abbo of Fleury attempting to reconstitute what they thought was the ancient programme of the Liberal Arts,[11] and turning to scientific texts at their disposal in their quest for new problems on which to exercise their minds. Computus began as simply the content available to fill the ancient categories of "arithmetic" or "astronomy," but when it came to be studied by men who were interested in solving problems, problems began to present themselves.

These problems—particularly the issue of the validity of traditional chronology, and of the discrepancies between the calendar and the astronomical phenomena—provided the momentum behind the quest of eleventh- and twelfth-century western thinkers for more sophisticated astronomical information. Computus was the door through which ancient and Arabic astronomy and mathematics entered the West, but what began as auxiliary sciences to computus ended by eclipsing their parent discipline. The change becomes rapidly visible in the form of the computus manuscript. The old "encyclopaedic" computus manuscript, where the calendar element dominates, with the subordinate fragments of extracalendrical material riding in its wake, never disappears. But beside it appears a new manuscript context for the computus. This type of manuscript, increasingly visible after the eleventh century, tends to anthologize computus materials (usually discursive texts rather than tables) into collections with a dominantly astronomical, mathematical, or medical character. In a sense, the "scientific anthology" computus manuscript represents an inversion of the early medieval situation where the computus contained the quadrivium. Now the quadrivium contains the computus, which has become a special or applied case of astronomy.

## 2. Medicine in the Medieval Computus Manuscript

As must be evident by now, computus manuscripts do not always—indeed only rarely—contain exclusively computus materials. They usually present themselves as anthologies, sometimes with the computus material as the controlling element (the "encyclopaedic" model), and sometimes with the computus as only one participant in a chrestomathy (the "scientific anthology" model). Medicine is a subject frequently found in association with computus, a fact that has inspired my project to describe some four hundred computus manuscripts, dating from the ninth to the fifteenth centuries, which contain medical materials, and to examine the contents of the medical texts, as well as their codicological and intellectual affinities to the computus materials.

This essay must perforce be more restricted in scope. First, I shall concentrate on manuscripts in which computus is the dominant element, and medicine one of the "penumbra" subjects; this is not the only kind of manuscript situation in which medicine and computus are found together, but it is the most promising environment for posing questions about why and how medicine attached itself to computus. Second, I will address only two of the many issues this material presents for our consideration: namely, what kinds of medical material are found in computus manuscripts, and how that material is related to its "host." I will do this by looking at the structure and contents of two exemplary manuscripts. The reader should understand, however, that I am proceeding this way only in order to furnish a concrete and realistic impression of the manuscript material and its possibilities; these two examples by no means exhaust the range of computus manuscripts or the medical materials contained within them.

Because the computus manuscript took shape in the early medieval period and first attracted medicine into its orbit at that time, the relationship forged between the two disciplines was strongly conditioned by the character of early medieval medical interests. First, these interests were decidedly untheoretical, an attitude inherited from the medicine of late Antiquity. Beccaria's study of early medieval medical anthologies reveals a very distinctive constellation of Galenic and Hippocratic texts, primarily concerned with humoral physiology, prognosis, regimen and herbal pharmacy.[12] This constellation dominates the content and determines the shape of pre-Salernitan medical manuscripts as a class;[13] it is entirely typical of early medieval medicine's concentration on a broadly cosmological explanatory context, and practical matters of preventative medicine and therapy. A second characteristic of early medieval medicine is that it was relatively unprofessionalized.[14] There were, to be sure, people who identified themselves as professional practitioners, but they did not monopolize interest in or access to medical knowledge. The Fathers of the Church considered medicine as a branch of secular learning comparable to grammar or astronomy, and therefore, like these other *disciplinae*, useful to Christian learning provided it was maintained in a subordinate role.[15] Indeed, they were deeply interested in the contribution medicine might make to understanding Biblical miracles of healing, as well as to a comprehensive allegorical interpretation of sin and salvation in terms of sickness and health. Moreover, care of the sick was an integral part of the practice of charity in Christian secular life and religious communities. In short, medical knowledge was viewed as a legitimate component of an early medieval cleric or monk's vocational education. Apart from the Scriptures and service books, the one volume that every cleric and monk had to have access to was a computus manuscript; hence medicine joined the other kinds of otherwise unclassifiable useful knowledge in the infinitely flexible "filing cabinet" of the computus manuscript.[16] The kind of medicine that found its way into the computus manuscript was the kind of medicine that purely medical manuscripts show us early medieval people were interested in: humoral physiology and pathology, prognostics, therapeutics, regimen, and herbal pharmacy. Within these broad categories, however, specific materials were selected for inclusion in computus manuscripts because they had some direct or analogous connection with time reckoning.

## 3. Reading the Contents of Computus/Medicine Manuscripts: Pal. lat. 485

MS Vatican City, Biblioteca Apostolica Vaticana Pal. lat. 485 is a ninth-century manuscript of German origin.[17] It is a clerical compendium, comprising prayers, expositions of the Mass and other sacraments, excerpts on ecclesiology and canon law, and penitential texts. The whole is prefaced by a computus section: since monitoring the liturgical calendar was a major responsibility of a priest—a responsibility stressed by numerous canon law provisions for preordination examinations in computus[18]—the inclusion of a computus anthology within a more general clerical anthology is understandable. The Pal. lat. 485 computus looks like this:

| | |
|---|---|
| Fol. 4r: | A table for locating the position of the Moon within the zodiac |
| Fol. 4v: | Computus notes (formula for finding the age of the Moon on January 1, reminders concerning leap day, mnemonic poem for finding the date of the *terminus a quo* for Easter) |
| Fols. 5r–5v: | Tables showing the age of the Moon on the first day of each month, and the weekday of the first day of the month, through the nineteen-year Easter cycle |
| Fols. 6r–11v: | Solar calendar with martyrology and computistical notes |
| Fols. 12r–13r: | A collection of lists useful for computus, of the standard type called *Computus graecorum* |
| Fol. 13r: | Prose text on the Egyptian Days |
| Fol. 13r: | *Lunare* for illness |
| Fols. 13v–14r: | Dietary and hygiene calendar for the twelve months of the year |

The last three items in our description are medical in nature. Each owes its inclusion to the fact that it concerns a medical application of the calendar. However, the three applications each have a very different character. For reasons that will become plain as the discussion proceeds, I will begin with the last item in the description, the dietary and hygiene calendar, and move backwards towards the first, the Egyptian Days.

## *3.1 Seasonal Time: The Dietary/Hygiene Calendar*

The dietary and hygiene calendar lists the months of the year, and provides advice as to the health regimen to be followed in each, e.g.,

> Incipiunt tempora pro sanitate corporis quae obseruari debeant.

> Mense martio. bibat dulce. usitet agramen. usitet radices. confectas manducare. asso balneo usitare. sanguinem minuare. solutionem non accipere quia frigores generat ipsa solutio.
>
> Mense aprili. sanguinem minuare. potionem bibere. carnes recentes manducare. sanguinem inter codinium minuare. calidos usitare. dolorem stomachi purgare. unguentos calasticos usitare. et si sic factum fuerit omnia membra sanare debent.
>
> Mense maio. calidum bibat. . . .
>
> [Here begin the times which ought to be observed for the sake of the body's health. In the month of March, one should drink sweet beverages, use pungent food and root vegetables, and chew one's food well. One should take sweat baths, undergo blood letting, but not take a purgative, because a purgative produces chills. In the month of April, undergo bloodletting, drink spiced wine and eat fresh meat. Blood should be let from the inside of the elbow. Eat warm foods. Purge stomachache, use soothing ointments, and if this is done, all the parts of one's body ought to be healthy. In the month of May, drink hot beverages. . . .]

Medical calendars of this type are very common in medieval manuscripts and have been studied extensively.[19] However, their frequent appearance in computus florilegia[20] has seldom been remarked upon, nor their specific relationship to the calendar defined. In fact, this relationship is rather problematic, for the medical calendar's ultimate sources have no direct connection to the twelve months of the Roman solar year. The ancient regimens that served as models for early medieval medicine, such as the ps.-Hippocratic *De salubri dieta* and *De victus ratione* or Anthimius' *De observatione ciborum ad Theodricum regem*, are closely coordinated to times, and like these medieval medical calendars, stress diet, bathing, bloodletting and herbal pharmacy.[21] But they are all seasonal, rather than monthly. The reorganization of these seasonal *regimina* into a monthly format can only have resulted from the early incorporation of such regimens into computus manuscripts.[22] In a computus manuscript, "penumbral" material tends to take the shape of the computus material in order to establish a secure foothold in the host manuscript. Neither the Roman calendar nor its Christian applications take any account of the seasons, and so the only element of a computus manuscript that can serve as a "hook" for a seasonal regimen is the solar year itself, of which the seasons are divisions. Hence the seasonal dietary comes to be modelled on, and in some cases, even physically inserted into the twelve-month Roman calendar.[23]

The original seasonal character of the ancient dietary was by no means obliterated, however. In one recension of the dietary and hygiene calendar,[24] whose unique manuscript witness is the computus florilegium in Paris, Bibliothèque Nationale nouv. acq. lat. 229, (s. XII), the old seasonal dietary is clearly visible beneath the superficial monthly organization. For example, in the entry for May, advice pertaining to the month slides gradually into admonitions concerning the summer season:

> Mense maio absinsthium et semen feniculi IIII. bibe et gamandream. de vena epatica minue. ad soluendum. accipe caputpurgia. oleribus frigidis utere. calidum bibe. nullius animalis caput uel pedes comedas quia tunc de caelo in rore descendunt uenena mala et de terra exurgunt deteriora. Ab VIII Idus Maii usque in VIII Idus Augusti crescit bilis amara. hoc est colera rubea. Utere rebus frigidis dulcibus et bene olentibus. quae facile digerantur. Frigidum bibe et aquosum. a uenere abstine quia virtus minuitur et stomachi debilitas ac tremor membrorum accidit. Ieiunia minime exequerere.
>
> [In the month of May drink wormwood with four grains of fennel, and wall-germander. Let blood from the hepatic vein. To purge oneself, take potion to purge the head. Use vegetables of a cold quality. Drink warm beverages. Do not eat the head or feet of any animal, because at that season poisons fall from heaven with the dew, and corruption arises from the earth. From May 8 until August 6 [i.e., the limits of the summer season according to Isidore of Seville, *De natura rerum* 7.5], bitter bile or red choler increases. Eat foods of a cold quality, sweet and fragrant, and which are readily digested. Drink cold and watered-down beverages. Abstain from sexual intercourse, because

> it diminishes one's vital forces; weakness of the stomach and trembling of the limbs result. Fast only a little.]

In some manuscripts the dietary calendar, even when it is actually inscribed on the margins of the solar calendar, retains a completely seasonal basis. This is the case, for instance, with Berlin, Staatsbibliothek 142 (s. XI$^2$); however, though the dietary regulations in this calendar are seasonal, the bloodletting and herbal pharmacy prescriptions are organized month by month.

Computus itself played a role in ensuring that this seasonal character was never wholly submerged. The astronomy necessary to understand the calendar was conveyed within a physics based on the four elements of earth, air, fire, and water, which were linked by pairs of shared qualities (heat and cold, moisture and dryness). This physics was incorporated into early introductions to computus, such as Isidore of Seville's *De natura rerum* and Bede's *De temporum ratione*, because the elements were believed to correspond to the four seasons. This in turn evoked the connection, fully developed in the ancient texts at the disposal of medieval writers, between the seasons and the four humors of the human body.[25] In short, the pedagogy of computus itself provided a niche for the humoral physiology that occupied such a large place in the early medieval medical interests. Hence Bede saw fit to devote considerable attention to this subject in *De temporum ratione*, Chapter 35, "On the Four Elements, Seasons, and Humors."

## *3.2 Astronomical Time: The 'Lunare'*

The next calendrical-medical element of Pal. lat. 485 we shall examine is the medical *lunare* on fol. 13r. A *lunare* is a list of brief prognostications or precepts for each of the thirty days of the synodic lunar month. *Lunaria* can apply to the general quality of the day, to bloodletting, nativities, decumbitures, and dream interpretation. One can find combined *lunaria*, or as in Pal. lat. 485, simple decumbiture *lunaria*, that is, prognoses of the outcome of an illness based on the age of the Moon on the day the patient fell ill.[26] *Lunaria*, like dietary and hygiene calendars, are very ancient, and have been documented in Greece, Egypt, and Babylon.[27] Like the dietary calendars, their presence in computus manuscripts is due to their obvious relationship to time. However, the kind of time they are related to is different from the time of the dietary calendars. Dietary calendar time is solar, seasonal, and sublunary time; time whose connection with the body is directly perceptible through changes of light, temperature, and atmospheric moisture; the outward manifestations of the elemental qualities. *Lunare* time is astronomical time, and the medical effects of changes in heavenly bodies like the Moon can only be inferred or deduced on the basis of a theory of celestial influence; they cannot be experienced directly and somatically, as can seasonal changes. Such effects were, to be sure, presumed to exist from ancient times, and were thoroughly integrated into the medieval conception of the relationship of the heavens to the body.[28]

The *lunare* in Pal. lat. 485 is typical of the early medieval conception of astronomical time in that the mechanism of celestial influence is not made explicit. Early medieval medicine believed unquestioningly in such influences, but was not yet equipped, and perhaps also unwilling, to develop a rationalized medical astrology. Chapter 28 of Bede's *De temporum ratione*, devoted to the influence of the Moon upon living organisms, is typical of the vague generalities of early medieval astrological medicine. Hence this *lunare* is an unvarnished list of bald prognoses, devoid of any explanation:

> Luna I qui ceciderit in infirmitatem. difficile euadit. Luna II cito resurgit. . . .
>
> [Whoever falls ill on the first day of the Moon will have difficulty escaping. Whoever falls ill on the second day of the Moon will soon be on his feet again. . . .]

Though medical astrology became much more sophisticated and diversified after the twelfth century, particularly with respect to calculating planetary motion, computus manuscripts tended to concentrate specifically on lunar astrological medicine. The computus, of course, was deeply concerned with the Moon, particularly in calculating its exact age, for on this hung the canonically correct dating of Easter. This concern opened the doors of the computus manuscript to the *lunare*, which found a secure home amongst its pages.

If the dietary and hygiene calendar links the medicine in computus manuscripts to the interests of early medieval medicine in general with humoral physiology, the *lunaria* reveal its fascination with prognosis. Prognostics played an important epistemological role in medieval medicine; given the limited ability of medieval physicians to actually cure disease, prognosis became the touchstone of the physician's claim to expert knowledge.[29] But just as the cosmology on which the computus rested shared a common ground (the elements and their qualities) with humoral medicine, so prognosis was as central a feature of the calendar, as it was of medicine. Conditioned by the need to project the dates of future Easters, Christian calendar lore is strongly oriented towards predicting future time. Certainly this prospective character attracted numerous texts of a prophetic or apocalyptic nature into the orbit of the computus. The calendar is also the locus of all kinds of prediction about the weather, a natural phenomenon closely linked in ancient medical tradition with health.[30] Other kinds of medical prognostica found in computus manuscripts will be discussed below.

## *3.3 Calendar Time: Egyptian Days*

The Egyptian Days are ominous calendar days.[31] Their character is determined not by the natural seasons, nor yet by the visible movements of the heavens, but by the arbitrary artifice of the Roman calendar. There are usually two (sometimes three) Egyptian Days each month; typically, the days are named by a count from the beginning or end of the month:

> Incipiunt dies aegyptiaci qui omni tempore seruandi sunt nec sanguinem detrahas nec medicamenta accipias. . . .
>
> Mensis ianuarius. alio die post kalendas et ubi facit dies XXIIII.
>
> Mensis februarius ubi facit dies IIII et dies XX et dies XXIIII. . . .
>
> [Here begin the Egyptian Days which ought at all times to be observed, lest you let blood or take medicine. . . . The

month of January: the second day after the Kalends and the twenty-fourth day. The month of February: the fourth day, the twentieth and the twenty-fourth. . . .]

No rationalizing explanation is offered for the Egyptian Days, though a few texts claim that they commemorate the days when God sent the plagues upon Egypt. Even a numerological basis seems wanting. They are a purely calendar prognostic, and the divisions of the Roman calendar are not correlated to seasonal or astronomical phenomena. Equinoxes and the solstices do not coincide with divisions of the months, and no heed is paid at all to the Moon. In short, while the Roman calendar's period is the solar year, its internal divisions are an arbitrary count of days.

The Egyptian Days, as simply "unlucky days," were carried over from ancient Roman calendars into their medieval progeny, and with them came a baggage of specifically medical admonition.[32] Rare is the calendar in a medieval computus manuscript that does not have the Egyptian Days inscribed against the date, or in the form of a poetic mnemonic at the head of each monthly page.[33] In not a few cases, discrete texts expounding the lore of the Egyptian Days are also found in computus manuscripts.[34]

Stepping back to look at the medical materials in Pal. lat. 485 as a group, we can see that the texts, similar in that they are all about medical applications of time reckoning, in fact deal with three kinds of time: seasonal time, astronomical time, and calendar time. These three kinds of time dictate the overall shape of medical material in almost all computus manuscripts, regardless of period. Under the rubric of seasonal time come not only the dietary and hygiene calendars, but discursive texts on seasonal indications for bloodletting,[35] and excerpts from the *Regimen sanitatis salernitanum* and its cognates.[36] By association, they bring in their wake more theoretical texts on the humors and complexions, and the relationship of these to the seasons and the elements,[37] or about other quaternity patterns within the human body, such as texts about the four regions (head, chest, belly, and viscera).[38] A good example of how these associations operate in practice is presented by London, British Library Arundel 334 (s.XV), an anthology of largely computistical and medical character.[39] A chronicle and calendar are followed by excerpts from the *Regimen sanitatis salernitanum* (fol. 22v), verses prescribing "quedam que in quibusdam signis anni vitanda sunt et utenda" [certain things which are to be avoided, or used, during certain zodiac signs in the year] (fol. 23r), the *Summa de sanitate regenda et conservanda* of ps.-Aristotle in the translation of John de Toledo (fol. 24), further hygiene texts, including "Qualiter homo se debet regere in quolibet mense tocius anni" [How a person should regulate his life during each month of the entire year] (fol. 89v), "Qualiter homo se debet regere in omnibus mensibus per annum" [How a person should conduct himself in all the months, throughout the year] (fol. 114v), and more excerpts from the *Regimen sanitatis Salernitanum,* "de quatuor complexionibus humani corporis quomodo se habent diversis temporibus anni" [On the four complexions of the human body, and how they are constituted at different times of the year] (fol. 116v).

When judicial astrology arrived in the West in the twelfth and thirteenth centuries via translations from Arabic and Greek sources, concepts of astronomical time underwent enormous changes. Its impact upon medicine was considerable, and it radically transformed the astronomical–time elements in computus manuscripts. Computists shifted their interests from predicting the date of Easter to predicting eclipses and conjunctions; the space formerly occupied by the martyrology in the calendar was usurped by the fifty-nine-year tables of lunisolar conjunctions and oppositions; and the planets joined the Moon and Sun as criteria for ordering one's regimen, or predicting the outcome of a disease. A typical late medieval medical-computus manuscript is Oxford, Bodleian Library Savile 39, written in England about 1436.[40] This slim volume (eleven folios) looks very much like a codex version of the folding almanacs described by Talbot,[41] which appear to have been especially popular in England. The Oxford manuscript contains a calendar with the fifty-nine-year table showing conjunctions and oppositions; a table of leap years from 1387–1507; explanatory texts about urinoscopy and bloodletting; a volvelle to show the longitude and phase of the Moon on any given day; a diagram of the influences of the zodiac signs; a circular diagram for urine inspection and a canon and table for lunar eclipses from 1392–1462. The accent is still on the Moon's influence over the body, but the discourse has moved away from generalities and bald prognostics towards more detailed and rationalized explanations and procedures for diagnosis and therapy.

Almost emblematic of the later medieval approach to astrological time and medicine is the *homo signorum*, or zodiac man,[42] a schematic drawing of the human body with the zodiac overlaid in Aries to Pisces sequence, from head to toe. Texts accompanying the zodiac man specify that on days when the Moon is in any particular sign, blood should not be let from the part of the body ruled by that sign; likewise, the organ ruled by that sign is likely at that time to be vulnerable to disease. The ancestors of this image are extremely ancient, and thoroughly astrological.[43] The zodiac man and its variant forms, such as the vein man, invade computus manuscripts after the fourteenth century.[44] New tables are created indicating the days of the lunar month appropriate for bloodletting,[45] and refinements are introduced, such as tables indicating the planetary rulers of each hour of the day,[46] also a relic of ancient astrology.[47] The relationship between the zodiac signs and the humors was also explored,[48] and a zodiacal parallel to the monthly health regimen appeared on the scene.[49] The impact of astrology on both computus and the medical materials found in computus manuscripts can only be alluded to here, but it is important to recall that it is essentially an elaboration of that concern for the medical implications of astrological time which, in much more primitive manifestations, is found in even the earliest manuscripts.

The concern with calendar time and its medical effects, on the other hand, hardly changed at all in the course of the medieval centuries. It essentially remained confined to the Egyptian Days and their variants. This stagnation was probably due to a certain medieval nervousness about the purely divinatory character of calendar prognostication; unlike astronomical medicine, it had no presumed natural basis, and smacked of superstition. It should be recalled as well that the Egyptian Days were carried over from the pagan Roman calendar. Even in some computus manuscripts, the arbitrary character of calendar medicine struck some observers as suspect. A group of texts in London, British Library Harley 2361 (fols. 10r–v) contains excerpts from St. Augustine's sermon 197 for New Year's Day, denouncing those who pay heed to lucky and unlucky calendar dates as no better than pagans; set in the midst of this is a diatribe against Egyptian Days, and another denouncing incantations against illness. Nonetheless, annual weather predictions—and by extension epidemiological predictions—based on the weekday or the weather on January 1 easily made the transfer from ancient astrology to the pages of the medieval computus manuscript.[50] Similar systems of arbitrarily ominous times for medical intervention, like the "three unlucky days," are part of this same constellation of calendar lore.[51]

A good example of this interface between prognostication, computus, and medical-calendrical interests is offered by the sprawling anthology in Oxford, Bodleian Library Digby 88 (England s. XV). Interspersed with calendar materials are some medical pieces, mostly of an astronomical time/prognosticatory complexion, but with some seasonal time elements. On fol. 14 there is a monthly dietary regimen, followed on fol. 15 by the Sphere of Pythagoras, a iatromathematical prognosticatory device discussed below. A note on the natural day (fol. 15v) and a text on the seven planets (fols. 16–23) are followed by another table for discovering whether a man or woman is likely to die (fol. 24). Another interesting constellation of texts begins on fol. 29r with verses on the four temperaments, followed on 29v with an English text on the influence of the zodiac signs. A bloodletting man follows on fol. 30r. After a group of texts on cosmology, thunder prognostications, the observance of Sunday, prognostications from the appearance of the Sun on Christmas Day, travel prognostications based on the appearance of the Moon, predictions of a woman's character from her physiognomy, chiromancy, critical days, and nativities, there is an extract from the computus treatise of John Somer on unlucky days (fol. 62v), and a table for bloodletting on each day of the lunar month (fol. 63). The next clutch of prognosticatory texts includes not only computus tables (fols. 77v–78, 81), computistical *argumenta* (fols. 80v, 82v), tables for moveable feasts (fol. 82r), and computus rules in verse (fols. 84–88), but also a circular diagram of the ages of man (fol. 83v), and the note on the three perilous days (fol. 77r). The manuscript concludes with more texts of a calendrical nature, prognostications of Antichrist (fol. 92r) and the Fifteen Signs of the Last Judgement (fol. 93v).

## 4. Reading the Context of Medical Materials in Computus Manuscripts: Oxford, St. John's College 17

The triad of dietary calendar, *lunare,* and Egyptian Days found in Pal. lat. 485 fits tightly into its calendar framework, both physically and intellectually. But the medical texts found in computus manuscripts can exist in varying degrees of affinity to the computistical core. In terms of understanding the messages encoded in the structure of these manuscripts, Oxford, St. John's College 17 (England, ca. A.D. 1110) offers a counterpart to Pal. lat. 485. In the synopsis of this manuscript presented here, the medical materials are in bold type:

1. Geometry problem (added in fourteenth or fifteenth century) fol.1r.
2. **Medical Anthology I (fols. 1v-2v)**
    a. **Treatise on four humors (fol. 1v)**
    b. **Treatise on bloodletting (fols. 1v–2v)**
    c. **List of herbs (fol. 2v)**
    d. **Prognostication of death (fol. 2v)**
    e. **Weights and measures (fol. 2v)**
    f. **Medical recipes (fol. 2v)**
3. Anthology of computus-related materials I (fols. 3r–15v)
    a. Abbo of Fleury: acrostic in honor of St Dunstan (fol. 3r)
    b. Grammar of numbers (fol. 3v)
    c. **Calendar prognostication (fol. 3v)**
    d. World ages (fol. 3v)
    e. Calculation of embolisms (fol. 3v)
    f. ***Lunaria* (fol. 4r)**

   g. Horoscope (fol. 4r)
   h. *Coena Cypriani* (fols. 4v–5r)
   i. Riddle (fol. 5r)
   j. Runic, cryptographic, and exotic alphabets (fol. 5)
   k. Riddle (fol. 5v)
   l. Demonstration of cryptographic techniques (fol. 5v)
   m. *Rotae* of Easter termini (fol. 5v)
   n. *Rota* of sunrises and sunsets (fol. 5v)
   o. *Mappa mundi* (fol. 6r)
   p. Feria table (fol. 6r)
   q. Degrees of consanguinity: tables and texts (fols. 6v–7r)
   r. Taxonomies of knowledge (fol. 7r)
   s. Byrhtferth's Diagram (fol. 7v)
4. Computus tables and texts I (fols. 8r–15v)
   a. Tidal *rota* (fol. 8r)
   **b. Sphere of Pythagoras (fol. 8r)**
   c. Computus tables (fols. 8r–12r)
   d. Byrhtferth's *Proemium* (fols. 12v–13r)
   e. Diagram of qualities of four elements (fol. 13r)
   f. *Computus graecorum* (fol. 13v)
   g. Computistical poetry and *lectiones*, glossed (fols. 14r–15v)
5. Calendar with martyrology (fols.16r–21v) includes **Egyptian Days.**
6. Computus tables and texts II (fols. 22r–37r)
   a. Tables keyed to calendar (fols. 22r–26v)
   b. Tables for Paschal computation (fols. 27r–34)
   c. Mathematics for computists (fols. 34v–35r)
   d. Lunar and solar time (fols. 35v–37r)
7. Cosmographical Anthology: Extracts from Isidore of Seville, Abbo of Fleury, and Macrobius (fols. 37v–40v)
8. **Iatromathematical prognostication (fols. 40v–41r)**
9. Mathematical Anthology: Texts on the abacus and on fractions by Hermannus Contractus, Gerlandus Compotista et al. (fols. 41v–58r)
10. Bede: scientific works (fols. 58v–123r)
   a. *De temporibus* (fols. 58v–61v)
   b. *De natura rerum* (acephalous; glossed) (fols. 62r–65r)

c. *De temporum ratione* (glossed) (fols. 65v–123r) Includes Chapter 35, **"De quattuor temporibus, elementis, humoribus."**

11. Helperic, *De computo* (glossed) (fols. 123r–135v)
12. Dionysius Exiguus (fols. 135v–157r)
    a. Letters to Petronius and to Bonifacius and Bonus on Paschal reckoning (fols. 135v–138v)
    b. Paschal tables with annals (St. John's 17 fols. 139r–143v, London, British Library Cotton Nero C.VII fols. 80–83—excised by Sir Robert Cotton in the seventeenth century—and St. John's 17 fols. 144r–155v)
    c. *Argumenta titulorum paschalium* (fols. 156r–157r)
13. Anthology of computus-related materials II (fols. 157v–159r)
    a. Texts on the zodiac (fols. 157r–v)
    b. *Sortes sanctorum* (fols. 157v–158v)
    c. ps.-Jerome on the grades of Roman society (fol. 158v)
    d. ps.-Jerome on fifteen signs preceding Last Judgement (fol. 159r)
14. Grammar Anthology: Texts on verbs and prepositional prefixes, orthography and prosody, and a précis of Priscian (fols. 159v–175r).
15. **Medical Anthology II (fols. 175v–177v)**
    **a. Recipes (fol. 175r)**
    **b. Charm for nose bleed (fol. 175r)**
    **c. Herb (fol. 175r)**
    **d. Classification and therapy of fevers (fol. 175r)**
    **e. Principles of pathology (fols. 175v–176r)**
    **f. Alphabetical list of herbs, with recipes (fols. 176r–b)**
    **g. Diseases and remedies (fols. 176v–177v)**

If Pal. lat. 485 illustrates a functional relationship between certain medical texts of an evident calendrical character, St. John's 17 exhibits analogous and symbolic, as well as functional relationships. These relationships are expressed by the physical positioning of the various medical materials within the manuscript.

To begin with, the self-conscious symmetries within this manuscript are very striking. Bede is the literal (as well as, apparently, the figurative) heart of the volume. His computus treatises are flanked by the two major tables of the computus and their satellites: on the one side by the calendar with its tables, and a group of "halo" materials (cosmology and mathematics), and on the other side by the Paschal tables with their attendant explanations by Dionysius Exiguus, and another group of "halo" texts (grammar). At each extremity of the codex we find, mirror-fashion, a group of computus-related materials, and a medical anthology.[52] Within these medical anthologies, the chosen texts echo one another: a text on humoral physiology and pathology, a herb list, and recipes. The treatises on the humors and on pathology at either end[53] are further linked by a common foundation on quaternities: the four humors, the four regions of the body, and so on. These quaternities form an analogous link to the four seasons of the year, as is evident from the fact that the Vindicianus text that underlies the text on fol. 1v of St. John's 17 is also the basis for Chapter 35 of Bede's *De temporum ratione*. It is interesting to observe that *De temporum ratione* occupies the exact centre of St. John's 17, and Chapter 35 is the midpoint of *De temporum ratione*. This thematic and structural symmetry might seem utterly fortuitous did it not recur in another computus manuscript, also made in England in the twelfth century, Durham, Dean and Chapter Library Hunter 100.[54] It suggests a vision in which time, the cosmos, and man are harmoniously connected by the shared structure of the four elements and their qualities. In medieval didactic diagrams, these interconnections of shared pairs of qualities knit the elements, seasons, and humors into a circle; the makers of St. John's 17 and Durham 100 seem to invite us to mentally join the matching ends of the manuscripts to form such a circle.

The texts on phlebotomy and taking medicine on fols. 1v–2r continue these themes by discussing the appropriate timing of these activities in relation to the seasonal ebb and flow of humors. The *prognostica* on fol. 2v is a list of the physiological signals of approaching death, which goes under the name of *Prognostica Galieni* or *Capsula eburnea*.[55] As we have seen, prognosis also has a functionally analogous relationship with the calendar. So also do the herb lists and recipes at either end of St John's 17.[56] The analogy here is not so much time, as the *measurement* of time. Computists were deeply conscious of the fact that their task was primarily one of measuring, indeed of measuring the immeasurable, and the symbolism of mensuration pervades computus manuscripts.[57] Recipes, like computus texts, are measurement literature, as are texts on weights and measurements, such as those on fol. 2v of St John's 17. Durham 100 draws these threads together by using a long extract from Isidore of Seville's *Etymologiae* 16.27 on weights and measures, ending with an anonymous text on pharmaceutical measures, to bridge its computus texts to its herb lists and recipes. Not surprisingly, both weights and measures and recipe collections are frequent denizens of computus manuscripts. The link between pharmacy and the calendar was reinforced by the notion that medicinal herbs had to be gathered at a specific time in order to maximize their efficacy.[58] In one computus-medicine manuscript, Cambridge, Trinity College R.7.23 (s.XIV), an appendix to a collection of English and Latin recipes arranges a list of simples according to the months. Not surprisingly, the most common kind of adventitious marginal addition to a computus manuscript is a medical recipe.

As we approach the calendar in St. John's 17, we move out of symbol and analogy and into more functional kinds of calendrical-medical texts: *lunaria* and Egyptian Days. Egyptian Days are also inscribed in the calendar proper, both as marginal annotations, and as calendar poetry at the head of each month.[59] Included in this section as well is the "sphere of Pythagoras" (also called the "sphere of Petosiris" or the "sphere of Apuleius"), a device that straddles the frontier between the astronomical time of the *lunare* and the arbitrary fortunetelling of the Egyptian Days.[60] The Sphere is a circular diagram, divided into an upper and a lower register; these registers may in turn be divided to make a total of four or six subregisters. The numbers 1–30 are inscribed in the various segments, apparently according to no plan. To use the Sphere, take the numerical value of the patient's name (using the formula A = 1, B = 2, etc.), add the age of the Moon on the day he fell ill, and divide the total by 30 (sometimes 29). Find the remainder in the Sphere. If it is in the upper register, the patient will live; if in the lower, he will die, and in the case of the four- or six-part Spheres, one can also determine the speed of his recovery or demise. Given the solicitude for symmetry we have already observed in St John's 17, it is no surprise to discover almost the same constellation of texts on the far side of the calendar, in the "iatromathematical anthology."

Two conclusions can be drawn from this reading of the structure of St John's 17. First, in the minds of the compilers, the physical distance of a medical text from the calendar denoted its functional distance; the farther from the calendar proper, the more theoretical the text. Second, the symmetrical structure of the manuscript encodes a metaphor about the "circularity" of computistical, cosmological, and medical knowledge—a sort of codicological transposition of the traditional diagram of the elements and their shared qualities.

Not every computus manuscript can be structurally "read" in exactly the same way as can St. John's 17, but almost all of them can be read. Their arrangement, like that of the Oxford manuscript, can reveal a logic and an aesthetic on the part of the compilers, over and above the logic governing the choice of medical materials for inclusion. This choice, on the other hand, is for the most part dictated by relevance of the medical material to one or more of the three kinds of time: seasonal, astronomical, and calendrical.

## 5. Conclusions and Directions

Within the confines of this essay, I have permitted myself to touch upon only a few salient points about computus manuscripts and their medical contents, illustrated by a very few examples. This has undoubtedly given the impression that this genre of source material is more uniform and tidy than it really is. I have had to subtract the "scientific anthology" computus manuscripts, as well as medical manuscripts containing *computistica*. These will all be dealt with in the final product of this project, as will the atypical medical materials, and the more eccentric or simply chaotic arrangements. Nonetheless, I think that these preliminary observations constitute valid guidelines for understanding the underlying logic of these manuscripts, and ultimately, the logic at work in the minds of the people who made them. Their conception of time, and their conception of the body in sickness and health, were both dominated by knowledge that was conveyed overwhelmingly through books. To a medieval reader, books were not just texts; they were texts incarnated in unique, particular sequences and shapes. It is in these incarnations that some concrete understanding of their experience of knowing about medicine must be sought.

## NOTES

*The research upon which this article is based was funded by grants from the Hannah Institute of the History of Medicine and from the Social Sciences and Humanities Research Council of Canada. Preliminary versions were presented in the fortnightly seminar of the Department of Social Studies of Medicine, McGill University, at the symposium on "Epistemology and the Scholarly Medical Traditions" organized by the Department in May 1992, and at the annual meeting of the Canadian Society for the History of Medicine in June 1992. I wish to thank the participants at all these presentations for their comments and suggestions.

1. These preliminary remarks on computus are a summary of my article "The Church, the World and the Time," in *Normes et pouvoirs à la fin du moyen âge*, ed. Marie-Claude Desprez-Masson and Regis Veyardier (Montreal: Ceres, 1989) 1–15. The reader should consult the references in this article, as well as in my chapter on "Chronology and Systems of Dating," in *Medieval Latin Studies: an Introduction and Bibliographical Guide*, ed. Frank A.C. Mantello and George Rigg (Washington: Catholic University of America Press, forthcoming) for a more extensive bibliography of primary and secondary works on computus. A useful survey of the history of computus, together with a thought-provoking appeal for a synthesis, is presented by Arno Borst in *The Ordering of Time: From the Ancient Computus to the Modern Computer*, trans. Andrew Winnard (Chicago: University of Chicago Press, 1993). Apart from Borst's volume, and a very concise sketch by O. Pedersen,

"The Ecclesiastical Calendar and the Life of the Church," in *Gregorian Reform of the Calendar. Proceedings of the Vatican Conference to Commemorate its 400th Anniversary, 1582–1982*, ed. G.V. Coyne, M.A. Oskin, and O. Pedersen (Vatican City: Pontificia Academia Scientiarum; Specola Vaticana, 1983) 17–73, the only general accounts presently available are found in prefatory material to editions of some computus treatises, in particular C.W. Jones's introduction to *Bedae opera de temporibus* (Cambridge, MA: Mediaeval Academy of America, 1943), Walter Emile Van Wijk's *Le numéro d'or: étude de chronologie technique suivie du texte de la Massa compoti d'Alexandre de Ville-Dieu* (The Hague, Nijhoff, 1936) and B. MacCarthy's *Annals of Ulster. Vol. 4, Introduction and Index* (Dublin, HMSO, 1901). The value of such introductions is restricted not only by their brevity, but by the fact that, as background to specific texts, they follow the development of computus only to the historical period where their text is situated. Bruno Krusch's admirable monographs are similarly confined in their chronological focus. His *Studien zur christlich-mittelalterliche Chronologie. Der 84jährige Ostercyclus* (Leipzig, Van Veit, 1880) deals with the period up to the sixth century, while his *Studien zur christlich-mittelalterliche Chronologie. Die Entstehung unserer heutigen Zeitrechnung*, Abhandlungen der preussischen Akademie der Wissen-schaften, Philosophisch-historische Klasse. Jahrgang 1937. 8 (Berlin: Akademie der Wissenschaften, 1938) is entirely concerned with Victorius of Aquitaine and Dionysius Exiguus. A. N. Zélinsky's essay on "Le calendrier chrétien avant la réforme grégorienne," *Studi medievali* ser. 3, 23 (1982): 529–597, despite its comprehensive title, concentrates for the most part on the medieval Russian calendar. Only a few of the major medieval texts on the computus have been edited, e.g., those of Bede, Rabanus Maurus, Alexander of Ville-Dieu, Grosseteste, and Bacon, as well as the vernacular treatises by Aelfric, Byrhtferth, Philippe de Thaon, and Nicholas of Lynn. Still awaiting modern critical editions are, to name but a few, the treatises of Helperic of Grandval (s. X), Garlandus (s. XI), Robert of Hereford (s. XI/XII), Cunestabulus (s. XII), Sacrobosco (s. XIII), John of Linières (s. XIV), and John of Gmünden (s. XV).

2. Only a few computus manuscripts have received thorough scholarly study. One is the subject of my University of Toronto doctoral dissertation *MS Oxford St John's College 17: A Medieval Manuscript in its Context* (1985). My unique forerunners in such an endeavour were G. G. Meersman and E. Adda, *Manuale di compoto con ritmo mnemotechnico dell'archidiacono Pacifico di Verona* (Padua: Antenore, 1966), a study of Florence, Laurenziana plut. 16, cod. 39. Numerous article-length treatments of other computus manuscripts are available, but the study of entire groups of computus manuscripts is the unique contribution of

Alfred Cordoliani, whose surveys of Spanish, Swiss, and British repositories, though far too numerous to list here, are the indispensible foundation for any future history of this science. Cordoliani has also published essays on individual computistical writers (e.g., Robert of Hereford, Garlandus, Dicuil, and Hermannus Contractus). Finally, he has provided essential, albeit not flawless, reference guides to much still unpublished computus literature in "Les traités de comput ecclésiastique du haut moyen âge (526–1003)," *Archivum latinitatis medii aevi* 17 (1942): 51–71, and "Contribution à la littérature du comput ecclésiastique au haut moyen âge," *Studi medievali*, ser. 3, 1 (1960): 107–137 and 2 (1961): 167–208.

3. These features figure prominently in the most important surviving manuscript version of the ancient Roman calendar, the so-called Chronograph of 354, or calendar of Furius Dionysius Filocalus, edited (without illustrations) by Theodore Mommsen, "Chronographus anni CCCLIIII," in *Monumenta Germaniae Historica. Auctores antiquissimi, 9: Chronica minora saec. IV-VII*, 1 (Berlin: Weidmann, 1892) 13–148; and (with illustrations) by J. Strygowski, *Die Calendarbilder des Chronographen vom Jahre 354*, Jahrbuch des Kaiserlichen Deutschen Archäologischen Instituts, Ergänzungsheft 1 (Berlin, 1888). The classic study is by Henri Stern, *Le calendrier de 354, étude sur son texte et sur ses illustrations*, Institut français d'archéologie de Beyrouth, Bibliothèque archéologique et historique, 55 (Paris: Geunther, 1953), recently revised and expanded by Michele Renée Salzman, *On Roman Time. The Calendar-Codex of 354 and the Rhythms of Urban Life in Antiquity*, The Transformation of the Classical Heritage 17 (Berkeley: University of California Press , 1990).

4. Catalogued by Atillio Degrassi, *Inscriptiones Italiae. XII: Fasti et elogia. Fasc. II: Fasti anni Numani et Iuliani* (Rome: Istituto poligrafico dello Stato, 1963): 284–298. See also Georg Wissowa, "Römische Bauernkalendar," *Apophoreton. Überreicht von der Graeca Halensis* (Berlin: Weidmann, 1903): 29–51; D. Foraboschi, "Manuali, calendari et trattati agricoli greco-romani," in *Studi in onore di Edda Bresciani*, ed. S.F. Bondì, S. Pernigotti, F. Serra, and A. Vivian. (Pisa: Giardini, 1985) 213–219.

5. On the naming of days in the Roman calendar, and the mnemonic features associated with this, see Agnes Kirsopp Michels, *The Calendar of the Roman Republic* (Princeton: Princeton University Press, 1967) 136. I elaborate on this subject in my essay on "The Roman Calendar: State Tradition and the Natural Order," in *Aufstieg und Niedergang der Römischen Welt* II.37 (forthcoming).

6. On Polemius Silvius's calendar and its sources, see Elizabeth Snowden Dulabahn, "Studies in the *Laterculus* of Polemius Silvius," Ph.D. diss., Bryn Mawr, 1987. Editions of ancient calendar poetry

include Emil Baehrens, *Poetae latini minores* (Leipzig: Teubner, 1883) 5: 349–356, and Alexander Reise, *Anthologia latina sive poesis latinae supplementum. Pars prior: Carmina in codicibus scripta* (Leipzig: Teubner, 1870) 1: 258–261. On ancient calendar poetry, see A.E. Housman, "Disticha de mensibus," *Classical Quarterly* 26 (1932): 129–136, and Salzman, *On Roman Time,* Appendix IV; for medieval calendar verse, see Paulus de Winterfeld, "Rhythmi computistici," *Monumenta Germaniae Historica. Poetae latini aevi carolini,* 4.1 (Berlin: Weidmann, 1899), and references cited in n. 59.

7. Jones, *Bedae opera de temporibus,* 75–76.

8. On the uninstitutionalized and vocational character of early medieval education, see Detlef Illmer, *Formen der Erziehung und Wissenvermittlung im frühen Mittelalter,* Münchener Beiträge zur Mediävistik und Renaissance-Forschung 7 (Munich: Arbeo-Gesellschaft, 1971); Pierre Riché, *Education and Culture in the Barbarian West,* trans. John Contreni. (Columbia, South Carolina: University of South Carolina Press, 1976).

9. An intriguing, if not entirely convincing reconstruction of how a computus manuscript would have been created and used as a "filing cabinet" in an early medieval monastery is proposed by Charles W. Jones, *Saints' Lives and Chronicles in Early England* (Ithaca, NY: Cornell University Press, 1947) 5ff.

10. Bede includes material on cosmology (e.g., ch. 34, "De quinque circulis mundi et subterraneo siderum meatu"), astronomy (ch. 25–29, on lunar eclipses and the various powers of the moon, including tides) and medicine. (Ch. 35 includes a discussion of the four humors of the human body.) Ireland would appear to be the place where this "halo" originated; cf. C.W. Jones, "The 'Lost' Sirmond Manuscript of Bede's Computus," *English Historical Review* 52 (1937): 210.

11. On Gerbert, see Uta Lindgren, *Gerbert von Aurillac und das Quadrivium: Untersuchungen zur Bildung im Zeitalter der Ottonen, Sudhoffs Archiv,* Beiheft 18 (Wiesbaden: Steiner, 1976). Concerning Abbo of Fleury's ambition to learn all the liberal arts, see Aimon of Fleury's *Vita Abbonis, Patrologia latina* 139, col. 390B–C, and G.R. Evans and Alison Peden, "Natural Science and Liberal Arts in Abbo of Fleury's Commentary on the *Calculus* of Victorius of Aquitaine," *Viator* 16 (1985): 109–127.

12. Augusto Beccaria, "Sulle tracce di un antico canone latino di Ippocrate e di Galeno," [pt. I] *Italia medioevale e umanistica* 2 (1959) 1–56 [pt. II], *Italia medioevale e umanistica* 4 (1962) 1–75, and [pt. III], *Italia medioevale e umanistica* 14 (1971) 1–21; see also Walter Puhlmann, "Die

lateinische medizinische Literatur des frühen Mittelalters," *Kyklos* 3 (1930): 396–401.

13. A cursory glance at the two standard repertories of early medieval medical manuscripts—Augusto Beccaria, *I codici di medicina del periodo presalernitano (secoli IX, X e XI)* (Rome: Storia e Letteratura, 1956) and Ernest Wickersheimer, *Les manuscripts latins de la médecine du haut moyen âge dans les bibliothèques de France*, Documents, études et répertoires publiés par l'Institut de Recherche et d'Histoire des Textes, 11. (Paris: Editions du C.N.R.S., 1966)—will confirm this impressionistically. Some illuminating observations on the typology of early medieval medical manuscripts are found in the the introduction to Groenke's monograph on dietary calendars (see n. 19); see also Peter Murray Jones, "Medical Books Before the Invention of Printing," in *Thornton's Medical Books, Libraries and Collectors: A Study of Bibliography and the Book Trade in Relation to the Medical Sciences*, 3rd ed., ed. Alain Besson (London: Gower, 1990) 1–29, especially his remarks on British Library Sloane 2839.

14. Nancy Siraisi, *Medieval and Early Renaissance Medicine* (Chicago: University of Chicago Press, 1990) 7–10.

15. Cf. H. Schadewaldt, "Die Apologie der Heilkunst bei den Kirchenvätern," *Veröffentlichungen der Internationalen Gesellschaft für Geschichte der Pharmazie*, n.s., vol. 26 (1965): 115–130; H.J. Frings, "Medizin und Arzt bei den griechischen Kirchenvätern bis Chrysostomos," Phil. diss., Bonn, 1959; M.E. Keenan, "Augustine and the Medical Profession," *Transactions of the American Philosophical Association* 67 (1936): 168–190; idem, "St. Gregory of Nazianus and Early Byzantine Medicine," *Bulletin of the History of Medicine* 9 (1941): 8–30; idem, "St. Gregory of Nyssa and the Medical Profession," *Bulletin of the History of Medicine* 15 (1944): 150–161; Karl-Heinz Leven, *Medizinisches bei Eusebios von Kaisareia*, Düsseldorfer Arbeiten zur Geschichte der Medizin 62 (Düsseldorf: Triltsch, 1987); G. Müller, "Arzt, Kranker und Krankheit bei Ambrosius von Mailand," *Sudhoffs Archiv* 51 (1967): 193–216; A. Nagel, "Die medizinische Anthropologie bei Ambrosius von Mailand," Med. diss., Düsseldorf, 1970; A.S. Pease, "Medical Allusions in the Work of St. Jerome," *Harvard Studies in Classical Philology* 25 (1914): 73–86; A. Peter, "Zu den medizinischen Anschauungen des Kirchenvaters Cyprian von Kartago," Med. diss., Berlin (East), 1969; W. Schwanitz, "Medizinisches bei Lactanz," Med. diss., Düsseldorf, 1975; K. Schweiger, "Medizinisches im Werk des Kirchenvaters Origines," Med. diss., Düsseldorf, 1983.

16. Interestingly, computists were frequently identified as having a special interest in medicine. For example, a computus treatise of A.D.

737 preserved in Berlin, Staatsbibliothek 128, refers to Dionysius Exiguus, the creator of the standard Paschal tables of the medieval West, as "vir in artemedica arte argutissimus." This is evidently a mistake for "in arithmetica arte," but the error is a revealing one: see Bruno Krusch, "Das älteste frankische Lehrbuch der dionysianische Zeitrechnung," in *Mélanges offerts à Emile Châtelain* (Paris: Champion, 1910) 234. The twelfth-century computist Ralf of Campo Longo was a physician, as was his fourteenth-century counterpart Simon Bredon: see C.H. Talbot, "Simon Bredon (c. 1300–1372), Physician, Mathematician and Astronomer," *British Journal for the History of Science* 1 (1962): 19–48.

17. Described in H. Stevenson, *Codices palatini latini,* t. I (Rome: ex Typographeo Vaticano, 1936) 155–158.

18. Cf. Charles W. Jones, "An Early Medieval Licensing Examination," *History of Education Quarterly* 3 (1963): 19–29.

19. Fifty different types of monthly medical calendar have been identified by Reiner Reiche, "Einige lateinischen Monatsdiätetiken aus Wiener und St. Galler Handschriften," *Sudhoffs Archiv* 57 (1973): 113–141. Nine common versions with their variants have been edited by Frank-Dieter Groenke, *Die frühmittelalterlichen lateinischen Monatskalendarien. Text—Übersetzung—Kommentar*, Diss., Institut für Geschichte der Medizin der Freien Universität Berlin, 1986. For further editions and commentaries, see Guy Sabbah, Pierre-Paul Corsetti and Klaus-Dieter Fischer, *Bibliographie des textes médicaux latins. Antiquité et haut moyen âge,* Centre Jean-Palerne, Mémoires 6 (Saint-Étienne: l'Université, 1987) 47–50. See also Jean Barbaud and Pierre Gillon, "Cinq calendriers diététiques provenant des manuscrits de la Bibliothèque nationale de Paris. Réflexions sur l'origine et la destinations de ces calendriers," *Actes du XXXe Congrès international d'histoire de la médecine. Düsseldorf, 31.VIII-5.IX 1986* (Düsseldorf: [Organisationskommittee], 1988) 179–185. Other studies of individual manuscripts include Pierre Bachofner, "Un calendrier enluminé de 1154, la Guta-Sintram de Strasbourg, et sa place dans l'histoire du medicament," *Revue d'histoire de la pharmacie* 179 (1963): 181–193; idem, "Notes sur les préceptes d'hygiène enluminés du Codex Guta-Sintram (1154)," in *Die Vorträge der Hauptversammlung der Internationalen Gesellschaft der Pharmacie e.V. während des Internationalen Pharmaziegeschichtlichen Kongresses in Rotterdam vom 17.–21. September 1963*, ed. Georg Edmund Dann (Stuttgart: Wissenschaftliche Verlags-Gesellschaft, 1965) 7–22 (Veröffentlichungen der Internationalen Gesellschaft für Geschichte der Pharmazie e.V, n.F., 26); idem, "Les préceptes d'hygiène enluminés du Codex Guta-Sintram (1154)," in *Le Codex Guta-Sintram (1154), manuscrit 37 de la Bibliothèque du Grand Séminaire de Strasbourg. Commentaires* (Lucerne and Strasbourg: Coptur,

1984) 157–165; Willy L. Braekman and M. Gysseling, "Het Utrechtse kalendarium van 1253 met de Noordlimburgse gezondheidsregels," *Verslagen en Mededelingen der Koninklijke Vlaamse Academie voor Taal-en Letterkunde* (1967): 575–635; and P. Alberdinck Thijm, *Kalendar en gezondheitsregels, getrokken uit het handschrift der Boekerij van de Hoogeschool te Leuven getiteld: "Liber orat. fland. M.S. . . ."* (Ghent: A. Siffer, 1893); A.G. Homblé, "Phlebotomiche en Hygiënische Voorschriften in XVe en XVIe eeuwse Handschriften en Kalendars," *Volkskunde* 72 (1971): 114–115. Studies of the texts of such monthly regimens include: Gerhard Eis, "Meister Alexanders Monatsregeln," *Lychnos* (1950–1951): 186–209, reprinted in *Forschung zur Fachprosa. Ausgewählte Beiträge* (Bern and Munich: Franke, 1971) 179–200. Karin Häfner, *Studien zu den mittelniederdeutschen Zwölfmonatsregeln*, Würzburger medizinhistorische Forschungen 3 (Pattensen/Hannover: Horst Wellm, 1975); Wolfgang Hirth, "Regimina duodecim mensium in deutschsprachigen Tradierungen des Hoch- und Spätmittelalters," *Medizinhistorisches Journal* 17 (1982): 239–255; Ria Jansen-Sieben, "Een Middelnederlands maandregimen uit der 14e eeuw," *Verslagen en Mededelingen der Koninklijke Vlaamse Academie voor Taal- en Letterkunde* (1971): 171–209; Gundolf Keil, "Das 'Regimen duodecim mensium' der 'Düdeschen Arstedie' und das 'Regimen sanitatis Coppernici,'" *Jahrbuch der Vereinigung für niederdeutschen Sprachforschung* 81 (1958): 33–48; idem, "Die Grazer frühmittelhochdeutschen Monatsregeln und ihre Quelle," *Fachliteratur des Mittelalters. Festschrift für Gerhard Eis*, ed. Gundolf Keil, Rainer Rudolf, Wolfram Schmitt, and Hans J. Vermeer (Stuttgart: J.B. Metzler, 1968) 131–146; idem, "Eine lateinische Fassung von Meister Alexanders Monatsregeln," *Ostbairische Grenzmarken* 4 (1960): 123–138, reprinted in *Medizin im mittelalterlichen Abendland* (Darmstadt: Wissenschaftliche Buchgesellschaft, 1982) 228–259; Agi Lindgren, "Eine altschwediche Fassung von '*Meister Alexanders Monatsregeln*,'" in *"gelêrter der arzenîe, ouch apotêker." Beiträge zur Wissenschaftsgeschichte. Festschrift Willem F. Daems*, ed. Gundolf Keil, Würzburger medizinhistorische Forschungen 24 (Pattensen/Hannover: Horst Wellm, 1982) 301–321; Ortrun Riha, *"Meister Alexanders Monatsregeln." Untersuchungen zu einem spätmittelalterlichen Regimen duodecim mensium mit kritischer Textausgabe*, Würzburger Medizinhistorische Forschungen 30 (Pattensen/Hannover: Horst Wellm, 1985); Karl Sudhoff, "Medizinische Monatsregeln für Aderlass, Schröpfen, Baden, Arzneigebrauch und Auswahl der Speisen und Getränke aus einer Pariser Handschrift des 14. Jahrhunderts," *Archiv für Geschichte der Medizin* 2 (1909): 136–139; and idem, "Ein Monats-Regimen," *Archiv für Geschichte der Medizin* 2 (1909): 434–436.

20. It is interesting to note that all the examples in Barbaud and Gillon's article (n. 19) are from computus manuscripts, though the authors do not mention this. To add but a few examples from across the medieval period, dietary calendars occur in Einsiedeln, Stiftsbibliothek 174 (s. $X^2$) fol. 68; Amiens, Bibliothèque municipale, Fonds Lescalopier 2 (s. XI); Munich CLM 14506 (s. XII) fol. 68; Munich CLM 17703 (s. XIII) fol. 96; Munich CLM 14706 (s. XIV) fol. 7; Munich CLM 13076 (1356) fols. 1, 26; Heiligenkreuz, Stiftsbibliothek 309 (s. XIV addition to s. XIII calendar); Munich CLM 5964 (s. XV) fol. 148r; Munich CLM 5595 (1432) fols. 35r and 49v; Erlangen, Universitätsbibliothek 496 (1453–1460) fol. 146v; Munich CLM 2777 (1458, 1469) fols. 32–37.

21. This is true of the many versions of the Hippocratic regimen-doctrine that circulated in the early medieval period, for which see Robert Joly, "Les versions latines du 'Regime' pseudo-Hippocratique," *Scriptorium* 29 (1975): 11–16. On ancient dietetics, see Ludwig Edelstein, "Antike Diätetik," *Die Antike* 7 (1931): 255–270, reprinted in *Medizinhistorisches Journal* 1 (1966): 162–174, and Georg Harig, "Die Diätetik der römischen Enzyklopädisten," *NTM* (1976): 1–15. For early medieval reworkings of this ancient material, see Karl Sudhoff, "Dieta Theodori," *Archiv für Geschichte der Medizin und der Naturwissenschaften* 8 (1915): 377–403, and "Lateinische Texte über den Rhythmus der Säftebewegung mit den Jahreszeiten, samt Nachtgleichen- und Sonnwends-Diätetik," *Archiv für Geschichte der Medizin und der Naturwissenschaften* 11 (1919): 206–211.

22. Barbaud and Gillon offer a similar hypothesis for the mutation of the seasonal dietary into a monthly dietary. Unfortunately, their argument is based on a series of errors. They argue that the monthly dietary was first propounded in ps.-Soranus's *Isagoge in artem medendi* (ed. in *Medici antiqui omnes* ch. 19, Venice, 1547), an argument that cannot be proven in the absence of a critical edition. However, they proceed to suggest that ps.-Soranus was brought back from Italy to England by Benedict Biscop in the seventh century, and thence incorporated into the *Computus vulgaris* printed amongst the works of Bede by Migne in *Patrologia latina* 90.762ff. But the *Computus vulgaris* in *PL* 90 is not a "text" at all, let alone a product of Bede's pen. It is simply a reproduction of the computus materials in the specific manuscript used by Noviomagus in his 1555 edition of Bede's computistical works; this edition was reprinted *tel quel* by Migne. "Computus vulgaris" only applies to the first table in this computus, a perpetual calendar invented by Abbo of Fleury (d. 1004), which bore a rubric whose first words were "Computus vulgaris [qui dicitur ephemerida Abbonis . . .]." In short there is no connection between Bede and the computus florilegium

printed in *PL* 90 as *Computus vulgaris;* hence the monthly dietary calendar printed in *PL* 90 cannot be traced back to ps.-Soranus, at least by this route.

23. Examples of the dietary and hygiene calendar being broken up and inserted onto the separate pages of a solar calendar include: Munich CLM 15909 (s. XIII/XIV) fols. 1ff.; Heiligenkreuz, Stiftsbibliothek 309 (fourteenth-century addition to a thirteenth-century calendar); Munich CLM 15719 (s. XIV) fols. 1ff.; Munich CLM 15176 (s. XV) fols. 1ff.; Munich CLM 15720 (s. XV) fols. 1ff.; Paris, Bibliothèque nationale Fonds Smith-Lesoeuf 39 (s. XVI in.) fols. 2vff.

24. Groenke's recension IVc, 199–207.

25. For a general overview of ancient humoral theory with special attention to these overlapping quaternities, see Erich Schoener, *Die Viererschema in der antiken Humoralpathologie, Sudhoffs Archiv,* Beiheft 4 (Wiesbaden: Franz Steiner, 1964).

26. On medical *lunaria,* see Christoph Weisser, "Das Krankheitslunar aus medizinhistorischer Sicht. Ein Beitrag zur iatromathematisch-astrologischen Fachliteratur des Mittelalters," *Sudhoffs Archiv* 65 (1981): 390–400; idem, "Zur Quellengeschichte des spätmittelhochdeutschen Krankheits-Speziallunars," *Studia neophilologica* 48 (1976): 325–329; and idem, *Studien zum mittelalterlichen Krankheitslunar: ein Beitrag zur Geschichte laienastrologischer Fachprosa,* Würzburger medizinhistorische Forschungen 21 (Pattensen/Hannover: Horst Wellm, 1982).

27. Weisser, "Das Krankheitslunar," 390. See also Max Förster, "Vom Fortleben antiker Sammellunare im englischen und in anderen Volksprachen," *Anglia* 67–68 (1948) 3–8, 35ff.; idem, "Die altenglishen Traumlunare," *Englische Studien* 60 (1925–1926): 62. See also Emanuel Svenberg, *De latinska lunaria. Tekst och studier,* Doktorsavhandlingar i latinsk filologi vid Göteborgs Högskola, Serie fr. o.m., 1926, XIII (Göteborg: Elander, 1936); idem, "Nya kollektivlunaria," *Eranos* 37 (1939): 75–83; idem, *Lunaria et zodiologica latina,* Studia graeca et latina Gothoburgensia 16 (Stockholm: Almqvist & Wiksell, 1963); and Erik Wistrand, *Lunariastudien,* Göteborgs högskolas årsskrift 48,4. (Göteborg: Elander, 1942). For examples from ancient Babylon, see S. Langdon, *Babylonian Menologies and the Semitic Calendars* (London: Oxford University Press, 1935) 73–82. Such lists are incorporated into Hesiod's *Works and Days,* and Pliny (*Historia Naturalis* 29.9) alludes to pocket almanacs "ad siderum motus ex ephemeride mathematica cibos dando horasque observando" which may have incorporated both the planetary hours and the position of the moon.

28. P. Saintyves, "De l'influence de la lune sur les maladies d'après les médecins astrologues des origines au XVe siècle," *Hippocrate* 2 (1934): 289–313, 405–433, 492–524.

29. Siraisi, *Medieval and Early Renaissance Medicine,* 133–138.

30. Stuart Jenks, "Astrometeorology in the Middle Ages," *Isis* 74 (1983): 185–210; Max Förster, "Beiträge zur mittelalterlichen Volkskunde," *Archiv für das Studium der neueren Sprachen und Literaturen* 120 (1908): 43–52 [on thunder prognostics]; 296–305; 128 (1912): 55–71 [on prognostication by wind and sunshine].

31. The fundamental studies of the Egyptian Days are Jules Loiseleur, "Les jours egyptiens. Leurs variations dans les calendriers du moyen âge," *Mémoires de la société des antiquaires de France* 33 (1872): 198–253, and R.S. Steele, "Dies Aegyptiaci," *Proceedings of the Royal Society of Medicine* 12 (suppl.) (1918–1919) 108–121; M. d'Alauzier, "Des jours néfastes au moyen âge," *Bulletin de la Société archéologique du Tarn-et-Garonne* 96 (1970–71): 79–80 (very summary and superficial); C. Cuissard, *Étude sur les jours égyptiens des calendriers,* Lectures et mémoires de l'Académie de Saint-Croix 5 (Orléans: E. Colas, 1882); P. Meyer, "Bribes de littérature anglo-normande," *Jahrbuch für romanische und englische Literatur* 7 (1886): 47–51; idem, "Les jours périlleux," *Bulletin de la Société des anciens textes français* 4 (1883): 93–95; idem, "Notices sur quelques manuscrits français de la bibliothèque Phillips à Cheltenham," *Notices et extraits des manuscrits de la Bibliothèque nationale* 24 (1891): 236–238; O. Södergard, "Notes sur les jours périlleux de l'année," *Neuphilologische Mitteilungen* 55 (1954): 267–271.

32. There is no doubt as to the *savant* character of the Egyptian Days, or their descent from ancient Mediterranean sources. Cf. Lynn Thorndike, *A History of Magic and Experimental Science* (New York: Columbia University Press, 1923–1958) 1:686; W.R. Dawson, "Some Observations on the Egyptian Calendars of Lucky and Unlucky Days," *Journal of Egyptian Archaeology* 12 (1926): 260–264; Max Förster, "Die altenglische Verzeichnisse von Glücks- und Unglückstagen," *Studies in English Philology, A Miscellany in Honor of Frederick Klaeber,* ed. Kemp Malone and Martin B. Ruud (Minneapolis: University of Minnesota Press, 1929) 258–277. Egyptian Days are found, for example, in the Chronograph of 354, and Petronius (*Satyricon* 30) describes an elaborate calendar attached to the doorposts of Trimalchio's atrium showing "lunae cursum stellarumque septem imagines pictas; et qui dies boni quique incommodi sunt, distinguente bulla notabantur." This would seem to have been a *parapegma;* for description of the *bulla* as a round-headed peg-marker, see Vitruvius 8.9–10. There may be a connection between the ancient astrologer's *partes damnandae* and Egyptian Days.

These *partes* (mentioned only in Manilius, *Astronomica* 4.408–501) are individual degrees of the zodiac which are excessively hot, dry, cold, etc. In the introduction to his edition of Manilius (Cambridge, MA: Harvard University Press and London: Heinemann, 1977, p. lxxxvii), G.P. Goold notes the hint of a pattern, in that the *partes* become more frequent the closer one gets to the end of a sign; in the case of Egyptian Days, they are clustered around the beginning and end of the month. Goold suggests (but does not demonstrate) that there might be some connection with the Egyptian calendar.

33. See n. 59.

34. Egyptian Days were by far the most popular, but by no means the only form of purely calendar-time prognostic. The seven days of the week, as much a calendar convention as were the Roman months, also attracted medical *prognostica:* see Christoph Weisser, "Mittelalterliche Wochentags-Krankheitsprognosen. Eine Gattung laienastrologisch-iatromathematischer Fachprosa," *'gelêrter der arzenîe, ouch apotêker': Beiträge zur Wissenschaftsgeschichte,* 637–653. For an example in a computus manuscript, see Vatican City, BAV Vat. lat. 687 (ca. A.D. 1400) fol. 123r.

35. Such a text appears, for instance, in Oxford, St. John's College 17 (see below), and in Berlin, Staatsbibliothek 142 (s. $XI^2$) fol. 54v: in both cases, the text is based on the ps.-Hippocratic *Epistola ad Antiochum.* Other examples of phlebotomy rules in computus-medicine manuscripts include Munich CLM 7038 (1417) fol. 217; Munich CLM 7650 (s. XIV) fol. 89r; Munich CLM 7688 (s. XV) fol. 28r; Munich CLM 8950 (s. XV) fol. 26r; Munich CLM 9921 (s. XII), with notes on bloodletting incorporated into the calendar, fols. 1–6; Munich CLM 13076 (1356) fol. 15 (this MS also contains bathing and dietary regimens); Munich CLM 14504 (s. XV) fol. 351r; Munich CLM 14622 (s. XV) fol. 163r; Munich CLM 14706 (s. XIV) fol. 1r.

36. See, e.g., Basel, Universitätsbibliothek F VII 12 (1445), a volume written in a single hand, contains, back to back, the *Regimen sanitatis Salernitanum* and the *Computus sacerdotalis* ascribed to Ludulphus de Wida. Erlangen Universitätsbibliothek 664 (1439) also combines computistical and astronomical material with a regimen, as does the "Mainauer Naturlehre" in Basel, Universitätsbibliothek B VIII 27; see Francis Brévart, "Die 'Mainauer Naturlehre.' Ein astronomisch-diätetisch-komputistisches Lehrbuch aus dem 14. Jahrhundert. Mit einer Quellenuntersuchung," *Sudhoffs Archiv* 71 (1987): 157–179. See also Munich CLM 5595 (1432) fol. 50r (excerpts from the *Regimen sanitatis salernitatum*); Munich CLM 7746 (s. XV) fol. 43r (*Regimen sanitatis*

*salernitanum*), 56r (anonymous regimen), and fol. 67r (Conrad of Eichstätt's regimen).

37. Some examples: Oxford, St John's College 17 and Durham 100 (discussed below); Vat. lat. 924 (s. XIII–XIV), verses on the four elements and the kinds of animal life; Erlangen, Universitätsbibliothek 475 fol. 47v (1516–1517), "Distinctiones quattuor complexionum"; Cambridge, Fitzwilliam Museum 167 fol. 77v–78r (ante 1487), with separate illustrations of the four temperaments; Munich CLM 19685 (s. XIV, XV) fol. 63 (on the relationship of the months to the complexions).

38. See, e.g., Oxford, St John's College 17, fols. 175v–176r (from ps.-Hippocrates, *Epistola ad Maecenatem*); Berlin, Staatsbibliothek 143 fol. 54v.

39. *Catalogue of Manuscripts in the British Museum. New Series. Vol. 1. Part 1. The Arundel Manuscripts* (London: British Museum, 1834) 99–100.

40. Falconer Madan and H.H.E. Craster, *A Summary Catalogue of Western Manuscripts in the Bodleian Library at Oxford*, vol. 2, pt. 2 (Oxford: Clarendon Press, 1937) 1110.

41. C.H. Talbot, "A Medieval Physician's Vade-Mecum," *Journal of the History of Medicine* 16 (1961): 213–233. There are many more folding almanacs than those enumerated by Talbot, the majority, though not all, being of a medical complexion: e.g., London, British Library Additional 17367 (s. XVI); London, British Library Additional 28725 (ca. 1460); London, British Library Egerton 2724 (s. XV); London, British Library Harley 3812 (s. XV); London, British Library Harley 5311 (s. XV); London, British Library Sloane 2250 (s. XV?); London, British Library Stowe 1065 (ca. 1482); London, Wellcome Institute Library 39 (s. XIV ex.); London, Wellcome Institute Library 40 (1463); Oxford, Bodleian Library Laud Misc. 753 (ca. 1387).

42. In general, see Charles West Clark, *The Zodiac Man in Medieval Medical Astrology*, Ph.D. diss., University of Colorado, 1979, and Harry Bober, "The Zodiacal Miniature in the *Très Riches Heures* of the Duke of Berry—its Sources and Meaning," *Journal of the Warburg and Courtauld Institutes* 11 (1948): 1–34.

43. Cf. Manilius, *Astronomica* 1, 453–465.

44. Some examples: Cambridge, Fitzwilliam Museum 167 (ante 1487) fol. 35v; Cambridge Trinity College R.15.18 (ca. 1400): 18 (with text); London, Wellcome Institute Library 40 (1463) fol. 7; Munich CLM 8950 (s. XV) fol. 6r; Erlangen, Universitätsbibliothek 664 (ca. 1439) fol. 35v; Paris, Bibliothèque nationale lat. 14668 (s. XV) fol. 195r. For a *rota* version of this material, see Oxford, Bodleian Library Ashmole 360.VIII

(s. XIV in.) fol. 159v. Often zodiac men attach themselves to a very venerable table for finding the position of the moon in the zodiac, e.g., in London, British Library Additional 41338 (s. XV). A similar pairing of zodiac man and lunar-zodiac table is found in the 1387 Catalan atlas (Barcelona, Bibliotheca Central) reproduced in Pedro Lain Entralgo, *Historia Universal de la Medicina*, vol. 3 (Barcelona: Salvat, 1972): 299.

45. See, e.g., Erlangen, Universitätsbibliothek 475 (1516–1517) fols. 41v-42v and 496 fols. 144v-145r, both s. XV; London, Wellcome Institute Library 39 (s. XV ex.) fol. 2.

46. See, e.g., London, Wellcome Institute Library 39 (s. XV ex.) fol. 7; London, British Library Additional 28725 (s. XV) fol. 1; London, British Library Additional 17358 fol. 2r; London, British Library Harley 3812 (s. XV ex.) fol. 5r; London, British Library Harley 5311 (s. XV) fol. 5r.

47. Dio Cassius (37.19) says that the legendary founders of astrology Petosiris and Nechepso devised the planetary week by assigning the hours, beginning with the first hour of Saturday, to each of the planets in descending order; the planet ruling the first hour of each day gave its name to that entire day. This system is also described by Vettius Valens, *Anthologiae* 11.1.10. The Potentia table (*Corpus Insciptionum Latinarum* 9.5808) designates the hours of Venus and Jupiter as *bonae*, those of Mars and Saturn as *noxiae*, and those of the other planets as *communes*.

48. See, e.g., in London, British Library Additional 15107 (s. XV), fols. 232v–233v: Aries enim est signum in complexione calidum et siccum . . . ; Munich CLM 4394 (s. XV) fol. 111r (on the four humors and the influence of the signs of the zodiac).

49. See, e.g., in St. Gall, Stiftsbibliothek 827 (1425–1428), fol. 263r, followed by the more usual monthly regimen on 263v; St. Gall Stiftsbibliothek 760 (s. XV) fols. 1–126.

50. See Bruno Assmann, "Prophezeihung aus dem 1 Januar für das Jahr," *Anglia* 11 (1889): 367 (from Cotton Vespasian D. XIV fol. 75v). Manilius associates prognostication of weather, epidemics, and war with January 1: *Astronomica* 1.401–406.

51. Cf. Gundolf Keil, "Die verworfenen Tage," *Sudhoffs Archiv* 41 (1957): 27–58. Examples of the inclusion of these "three unlucky days" for bloodletting or taking medicine include Oxford, Bodleian Library Digby 88 (s. XV) fol. 77r, Vatican City, BAV Vat. lat. 644 fol. 77 (s. XI additions to a s. X MS), and London, British Library Arundel 332 (s. XIII), a clerical anthology, with a substantial section on computus,

astronomy, and algorism running from fols. 32r–73v. Prefacing this section on fol. 31v is a note on the three unlucky days for bloodletting. See also Oxford, St. John's College 17, discussed below.

52. These medical anthology texts were presented and edited, albeit imperfectly, by Charles Singer in two versions of an essay published almost simultaneously in two journals: "A Medical Compendium of the First Half of the Twelfth Century," *Bulletin of the Medical History Society of Chicago* (January 1917): 43–96, and in a somewhat revised form as "A Review of the Medical Literature of the Dark Ages, with a New Text of About 1110," *Proceedings of the Royal Society of Medicine* 10 (1917): 107–160.

53. The text on the four humors on fol. 1v is a close paraphrase of Vindicianus Afer's *Epistula ad Pentadium Nepotem*; that on pathology at the back of the volume is *quasi verbatim* from the *Epistula Hippocratis ad Maecenatem*.

54. The present arrangement of the gatherings in Durham 100 is not the original one: see Fritz Saxl and Hans Meier, *Catalogue of Astrological and Mythological Illuminated Manuscripts of the Latin Middle Ages. Vol. 3: Manuscripts in English Libraries*, ed. Harry Bober (London: Warburg Institute, 1953): 441–447. Reconstituted, it looks like this:

-Anonymous text on the four humors

-Excerpts from Isidore of Seville's *Etymologiae* on medicine (bk. 4), on man and his parts (bk. 11) on pharmacy (bk. 17), plus further notes on medicinal herbs from Ambrose and Rabanus Maurus

-computistical core, including solar calendar, Paschal tables, additional tables and texts

-texts on music by Boethius and Guido d'Arezzo

-Helperic's *De computo*, plus extracts from Bede's computus treatises

-texts on astronomy by Abbo of Fleury, Isidore of Seville, etc.

-extracts from Isidore on weights and measures (bk. 6, ch. 23) ending with an anonymous text on pharmaceutical measurements

-herb list

-medical recipes

-a second herb list, with remedies

-further recipes and medical charms

-cautery diagrams

St. John's 17 and Durham 100 might also be compared to Vatican City, BAV Reg. lat. 258 (England? s. XIII in.) The character of this codex is curiously coherent, despite its superficial air of being a miscellany. Its core is a bestiary. Flanking it on both sides are two groups of short texts combining moral, theological and liturgical themes with miscellaneous natural history, particularly astronomy/computus and anthropology/medicine. Wilmart, in his catalogue of the Reginenses manuscripts (*Codices Reginenses latini*, T.II, Codd. 251–500 (Vatican City: Biblioteca Apostolica Vaticana, 1945): 24–26) claims that this codex is acephalous, but I can detect no evidence for this view. The fact that the "parenthesis" structure, where a distinctive core is framed at both ends by a constellation of resonant materials, appears in other manuscripts, would argue for its integrity. As a phenomenon of medieval book aesthetic, it merits further investigation.

55. See Vivian Nutton, "Prognostica Galieni," *Medical History* 14 (1970): 96–100.

56. On the importance of texts on weights and measures in medical manuscripts, see Henry Sigerist, "Masse und Gewichte in den medizinischen Texten des frühen Mittelalters," *Kyklos* 3 (1930): 439–444.

57. For a fuller discussion of this topic, see my article "Images of Order in the Medieval Computus," in *ACTA XIV: Ideas of Order in the Middle Ages*, ed. by Warren Ginsberg (Binghamton: State University of New York Press, 1990) 45–67.

58. See Ernest Wickersheimer, "Epistola Ypocratis ad Alexandrum de tempore herborum," *Janus* 41 (1937): 145–152; idem, "Nouveaux textes médiévaux sur le temps de cueillette des simples," *Archives internationales d'histoire des sciences* 3 (1950): 342–355; idem, "Sur le temps de cueillette des simples. Deux textes inédits," in *Homaje a Millás-Vallicrosa* (Barcelona: Consejo Superior de Investigaciones Científicas, 1956) 2.523–527.

59. The poem on the Egyptian Days, "Iani prima dies et septima fine timetur . . . Dat duodena cohors septem inde decemque december," is edited in Migne, *Patrologia latina* 90.761ff. and 90.956, and by John Hennig, "Versus de mensibus," *Traditio* 11 (1955): 83. The poem could be reproduced as a whole, or broken up into individual lines, one line per month, in a calendar. Such calendar poetry forms a genre unto itself: see Karl Strecker, "Zu den komputistischen Rhythmen," *Neues Archiv* 36 (1911): 317–342, and Günter Bernt, *Das lateinische Epigramm im Übergang von der Spätantike zum frühen Mittelalter*, Münchener Beiträge zur Mediävistik und Renaissance-Forschung 2 (Munich: Arbeo-Gesellschaft, 1968): 286–294. The Egyptian Days poem is one of the most frequently encountered of such poems in the calendars of computus manuscripts.

60. On the Sphere of Pythagoras, see Ernest Wickersheimer, "Figures médico-astrologiques des IXe, Xe et XIe siècles," *Janus* 19 (1914): 157–177; Charles Singer, "Early English Magic and Medicine," *Proceedings of the British Academy* 9 (1919–1920) 341–373; Henry Sigerist, "The Sphere of Life and Death in Medieval Manuscripts," *Bulletin of the History of Medicine* 11 (1942): 292–303, and Ernst Reiss, "Nechepsonis et Petosiridis fragmenta magica," *Philologus*, Suppl. 6 (1891–1893): 325–394. Similar forms of medical divination based on the numerical values of the letters of the patient's name, and prognosticating according to oppositions of life/death, swift recovery/slow recovery, are practiced to this day by Christian *debdera* (itinerant healers) in highland Ethiopia: see Allan Young, "Order, Analogy and Efficacy in Egyptian Medical Divination," *Culture, Medicine and Psychiatry* 1 (1977): 183–199, esp. 187–189, and Marcel Griaule, "Notes sur l'arithmomancie ethiopienne," *Journal de la Société des africanistes* 4 (1934): 25–31.

# Manuscript Sources for Birth Control

*John M. Riddle*

One way to learn what medieval people knew about chemical means of birth control is to explore the way they translated technical concepts into their own language. Manuscript sources are indispensable in finding this data. When manuscript evidence is combined with scientific data about the chemical drugs they were taking, the conclusion is that medieval people were aware of effective means to control births and regulate family sizes.

Rue (*Ruta graveolens* L.) is a perennial herb that grows to about three feet and possesses bluish green flowers. Some people do not like its aroma. The popular *Reader's Digest* herbal book, *Magic and Medicine of Plants* (1986) says that it was used as an antispasmodic, anthelmintic, and emmenagogue. In parentheses, the editors of the herbal defined an emmenagogue as "an agent that brings on menstruation" (286).

The classical and medieval medical texts in Greek and Latin frequently referred to rue in similar terms. For example, Constantine the African's *De gradibus* found in Munich MS lat. 267 (s. xiv, fol. 128v) has "menstrua provocat." Soranus, Galen, and other medical writers gave greater detail, but there appears to be a contradiction in their accounts. Pliny and Galen called rue an abortifacient.[1] Soranus wrote that rue was an oral contraceptive.[2] Inexplicably, however, the foremost authority on drugs, Dioscorides (fl. first century A.C.E.) omitted any such reference to rue's alleged birth control property.[3] However, some scribe who was copying Dioscorides, was mindful of the inexplicable omission. The scribal alteration is first found in Paris Bibliothèque nationale Ms gr. 2179, written in the ninth century. Added to the text was the following: (κινεῖ δὲ καὶ καταμήνια, τὰ δὲ ἔμβρυα φθειρει)."[4] Translated: Rue "brings forth the menstrua and aborts an embryo." Neither the Greek nor the Latin made the distinction that we do between an embryo and a fetus, so we must live with the ambiguity. There was no mistake about the meaning: Rue was a birth control agent. Subsequently, a number of Dioscorides's manuscripts included the emendation so a reader might know that rue was not only an emmenagogue but it was also an abortifacient.

As the *Reader's Digest* editors explained, an emmenagogue is an agent that provokes menstruation. Unexplained by the editors is the fact that the action occurs regardless of whether a fertilized embryo is present. The equation of an emmenagogue with an abortifacient even escaped the cognizance of many physicians in the nineteenth century when abortion was made a criminal offense.

Historians have regarded the appearance of oral contraceptives and early-term abortifacients in medical documents as magic, superstition, or ineffectual nonsense. They believed that only in the modern era, notably the mid-1950s when the "pill" was marketed, was there such knowledge. It was not until the 1960s that studies of such botanical agents began to be reported in Indian and Chinese medical and pharmaceutical journals. Western scientists now are reexamining their previous skepticism that such agents actually affected fertility and so must historians follow their science colleagues and attribute more credibility to their documents. After all, the medical documents are filled with the prescriptions. The literature is filled with anecdotal evidence. The legal and theological evidence, notably that examined by John Noonan, contains copious references to the legality and morality of chemical abortions and, to a lesser degree, contraceptives.[5]

Perhaps most important, the demographic evidence in classical antiquity and the medieval period is certain: Somehow premodern peoples engaged in practices that suppressed population growth and, at times, produced declines.[6] Restraint, potentially nonfertile intercourse procedures, and infanticide are the means most prominently proposed. Most notable are the data presented by David Herlihy about late medieval Tuscan women who limited family size to a few children even though they had scores of years of pregnancy vulnerability.[7] Moreover, the number of children per family varied according to economic status, with the poorer families having fewer children than the more wealthy ones.

Before exploring what medieval peoples knew and how they knew it, let us explore rue's pharmacology as presently known. Today rue is employed as an abortifacient in the form of a tea throughout Latin America and among the Hispanic population of New Mexico. It is employed in the traditional medicine of India for the same purpose.[8]

In 1989, Chinese investigators explored the antifertility effects of rue, administering chloroform extracts of the whole rue plant in daily oral doses of 0.8 to 1.2 grams per kilogram to female rats over the first eight to ten days of pregnancy. The extracts reduced the number of pregnancies in the experimental group by 20 to 75 percent (depending on the potency of the extract administered).[9]

Rue belongs to the botanical family, Rutaceae, which includes several plants that produce antifertility agents. Chinese scientists have studied the active substance in another Rutaceae species. The substance, called *yuechukene* and extracted from the plant *Murraya paniculata* (var. *Murraya sapientum* L.), has been reported to be 100 percent effective in preventing pregnancies in rats when administered orally at doses of 2 milligrams per kilogram during the first six days of pregnancy, or as a single dose of 3 milligrams per kilogram on the first day after coitus.[10] This study shows that the action was that of a contraceptive in that it prevented implantation. Therefore, the apparent contradiction found in the sources probably is not at variance with the reality as we know it. It is interesting that another Rutaceae species, *Pilocarpus jaborandi* Homes, produces a cholinergic agent called pilocarpine that has been given to horses to induce abortion.[11]

Did classical and medieval people know that if an emmenagogue (menstrual regulator) was taken when the woman was pregnant, she would terminate pregnancy? Both published texts and manuscripts provide interesting evidence that they knew that a menstrual regulator acted as a birth control agent as well.

Pliny the Elder, who opposed abortion, said that rue promoted menstruation, brought away the afterbirth, and expelled a dead fetus (or embryo).[12] In a dissertation in 1927, Johannes Fischer showed that Pliny, like Dioscorides, commonly used the concept of expelling a dead fetus as meaning an abortion or producing a miscarriage.[13] Indeed Pliny himself acknowledged the meaning in reference to rue when, in another section of the *Natural History*, he wrote a precautionary note: "Pregnant women must take care to exclude rue from their diet for I find that the fetus [or embryo] is killed by it."[14]

At the end of the Middle Ages in a manuscript written in 1493, now at the College of Physicians in Philadelphia, there is a recipe titled "Ad menstrua provocanda," which is taken orally "nisi pregnans sit."[15] At the beginning of the Middle Ages, Gargilius Martialis, whose work otherwise contains no birth control suggestions, wrote this about rue:

> Some very foolishly declare the damage rue causes: that it inhibits, debilitates the generative seed, and kills embryos in the womb. By itself it does not bring these results; they are due to the people who employ it without considering its strength, its dosage, or the circumstances.[16]

Many of the Latin translations of Greek medical works were done about the fifth and sixth centuries. During this period, Dioscorides's *Materials of Medicine* was translated anonymously by someone probably in the Ravenna area of Italy. The translator exhibited no inhibitions in dealing with birth control and, by his choice of words, revealed that he understood the subject matter.

Dioscorides said of the bark of white poplar, "ἱστορεῖται δὲ καὶ ἀτόκιοζ εἶναι" for "it is reported to be a contraceptive (ἀτόκιοζ)."[17] As found in Munich manuscript 337 (tenth century), the unknown Latin translator wrote: "Hanc multi asseverant, quod bibita . . . generare non permittit," or, "It is asserted by many that, drunk, it does not permit one to generate."[18] Clearly, this is not so much a translation as it is an informed interpretation. Similarly the next line in Dioscorides's

Greek reads, "τὰ φύλλα δὲ πινόμενα μετὰ (τὴν) κάθαρσιν σὺν ὄξει τὸ αὐτὸ δρᾶν λέγεται," meaning, "its leaves after the dirty period (i.e., menstruation), it is said, clean greater than the other (i.e., the bark)."[19]

The Latin translator found in Munich 337 handles the complex Greek far more easily than the original with "Folia eius bibita post purgationem menstruorum simili modo minime conceptum admittit," or, "Its leaves drunk after the menstrual purge allows conception to take place to a less effective degree than the bark."[20] Evidently the early medieval translator was familiar with the medical concept of contraceptive (as understood by the time period) because the translation, in this case, is more clear and explicit than the original Greek.

Elsewhere in the same work, where the Greek text said, "[Pepper] drives out the embryo; if applied as a suppository after intercourse, it prevents conception,"[21] the Latin translation reads: "It is thought after coitus that it kills by poisoning; let it be applied after intercourse into the genital area."[22] To be sure, the "translation" was not a literal rendering of words but, again, an interpretation. It was not that the translator did not know his/her languages; s/he said, as, when s/he translated Dioscorides on death carrot: "ἔμβρυα φθείρει (it aborts an embryo)" into "abortum facit (it makes an abortion)."[23]

In the Latin translation of Oribasius's work, there is a discussion about abortions (ἐκβάλλοντα ἔμβρυα),[24] where many of the plants (rue, dittany, birthwort, myrrh, pennyroyal, juniper, cypress, asarus, artemisia, and iris) are referred to, but rather than abortifacients they are called emmenagogues (e.g., "purgat menstruam").[25] A generalization that I initially made, but subsequently repressed, was that the Middle Ages, because of religious and theological positions on birth control, generally disguised abortifacient agents as emmenagogues.[26] While there was during the Middle Ages a *gradual* trend away from explicit mentioning of oral contraceptives and abortifacients, there never was a period during the Middle Ages when birth control agents were not recorded.

It is not always true, however, that the Latin texts of the early Middle Ages (when the Latin translation of Oribasius was done) reflect a reluctance to mention specific data about abortions. For example, the Latin herbal known as Pseudo-Dioscorides's *Ex herbis femininis* (composed during the sixth century) has an explicit statement, not found in classical sources, for the plant ploughman spikenard: "Its juice, placed on wool and introduced to the genital region, causes an abortion in a pregnant woman."[27] In a rough screening laboratory study reported in an Indian journal in 1966, spikenard was found to have an antiovulatory activity. There are modern folk-medicine reports that spikenard is used as an emmenagogue.[28] The early medieval herbal was correct when it said that spikenard caused an abortion.

A near consensus about the drugs is seen in the Latin *Synopsis* of Oribasius (which was also done in the fifth or sixth century). In the discussion of menstrual regulators and emmenagogues, a number of agents are mentioned: "beaten wormwood, pennyroyal, century plant, thyme, rue and *others which have those qualities*."[29] Clearly, the author thought that the reader would know what the remaining plants were. Examples: for cabbage stalks, "purgationem feminis . . . emortuos pellit;" for rue, "feminarum etiam purgationes secundasque etiam emortuos partus."[30]

Not only did the knowledge of birth control agents continue during the Middle Ages but manuscript sources reveal that it was extended. An Old English herbal, primarily translated from the herbals by Pseudo-Apuleius and Pseudo-Dioscorides, the earliest manuscript of which is ninth century, said that nettle (*Urtica* sp.) was an emmenagogue.[31] This information was not in the sources employed. The information came from another textual source or as a contemporary emendation from information derived from folklore. A recent animal test of *Urtica dioica* L. showed a 33 percent activity in preventing implantation in albino rats, and it is known in medical reports as an abortifacient.[32]

Tansy (*Tanacetum vulgare* L.) is a familiar plant to most of us, a hardy aromatic perennial with small, buttonlike flowers. It is indigenous to Europe and brought to North America, it escaped from gardens and now grows wild as well. We know the plant and the Greeks and Romans must have also (even though it prefers climates cooler than Athens and Rome). There is no word for tansy in classical Latin or Greek or, at least, there is no word identified in the extant literature. Therefore, it is of interest that the first surviving mention of tansy appears in the *Physica* of St. Hildegard of Bingen. The manuscript indicates, however, that the text was an emendation.[33] There is no doubt that Hildegard knew the plant, calling it by its German name, *reynfan*. The emendation simply says: "Mulier ergo quae obstrusa menstrua patitur, et inde dolet, accipiat tanacetum (Women, therefore, who suffer from retention of the menstrua and are ill from it, take tansy)."[34] Note that the emendator employed the Latin term, *tanacetum*. In medicine today, tansy is known as an abortifacient, technically, an ecbolic.[35]

Although Hildegard lived in a cloister, she was worldly enough to know of seven plants that she said were emmenagogues. She did not rely primarily on texts, simply because she did not know the Latin word for many of the plants, and hence used a German common name. She must have learned from her friends, neighbors, and, of course, the sisters. She knew that when she recommended a menstrual stimulator, pregnancy also might be terminated. Concerning the plant that she called *haselwurtz*, which we call asarum (*Asarum europaeum* L.), she made it clear, "A pregnant woman will eat it, either on account she languishes (*morietur*), or she aborts an infant with a danger to her body, or if she has not had a menstrual period for a time period so that it hurts."[36] Concerning the plant she called *metra*, our feverfew chrysanthemum (*Chrysanthemum parthenium* L.), she simply wrote that women who suffered from menstruation, should eat it because *menstrua educit*.[37] She was much more specific about *hirtzswam* or oleaster (*Elacagnus angustifolia* L.): "It makes an abortion to a pregnant woman with a danger to her body, should she eat this plant."[38]

Hildegard must have been learning from the common folk around her convent, because we can find no texts from which her information comes. Moreover, had she known the Latin names for many of the plants, she would have used them just as she did for the ones she knew. When we rely mostly on texts, it is difficult to learn what the common folk did. Writing between 1307 and 1311, Peter of Padua wrote a gloss as marginal note beside the entry for *asarus* in the Latin text of the Alphabetical

Dioscorides. In it he commented that the herb is taken by uninformed people before coitus.[39] Here we have an explicit statement about popular use of what is presumably a birth control drug. In addition to the testimony from the text, we now have evidence from scientific and medical studies that asarum has abortifacient qualities.[40]

The issue is whether ancient and medieval people were aware that, when emmenagogues or menstrual regulators were taken, they could also be used as birth control agents. Artemis, the goddess of women and woodland, and the protector of childbirth, gave her name to a group of shrublike plants that can grow to about four feet. In classical times, artemisia was said to protect against the pangs of childbirth, although no one stated whether it did so by preventing or terminating a pregnancy, or by some other means. During the Roman Empire, both Soranus and Dioscorides reported that physicians prescribed species, wormwood or *Artemisia absinthium*, as an abortifacient drug.[41] Other ancient medical authorities classified wormwood as an abortifacient and as an emmenagogue.[42]

Artemisia has not been forgotten. Again, a report from the *Reader's Digest* book *Magic and Medicine of Plants* says that artemisia provokes menstruation.[43] There is modern scientific support for the abortion-inducing effects of the drug. Animal studies over the past twenty years have reported that wormwood has delayed the production of estrus and ovulation and interfered with implantation. One study indicates that wormwood has an effect on males as well—interfering with spermatogenesis.[44]

Sometime in the late eleventh century, the central Middle Ages' most popular herbal was written in Latin verse. This is Macer's *De virtutibus herbarum*. In my opinion, the author, who often is identified as Odo of Meung, was Marbode, Bishop of Rennes (1035–1123). In any case, the first of the seventy-two herbs listed was artemisia. Macer or Marbode explained that the herb was named after the goddess, Artemisia, Diana to the Romans, who discovered "that it cures mainly female ailments." He wrote, "It stimulates menstrua and, whether drunk or applied, it produces an abortion."[45]

In the late twelfth or early thirteenth century there may have lived in or around Salerno a woman physician named Trotula. Among the various versions of the gynecological treatise allegedly written by her, there is a section on emmenagogues. The advice given is that, if one suffers from retention of the menses, one should drink artemisia in wine and take baths. If this proves ineffective, the work prescribes a number of herbs, such as the death carrot, to be taken with artemisia.

The same pattern repeats itself with pennyroyal (*Mentha pulegium* L.). Macer's herbal: "If a pregnant woman takes this herb often, she will abort./ It draws off the menses when taken with tepid water."[46] The ingestion of pulegone, the active substance in pennyroyal, has been shown in recent studies to induce abortions in women and in animals. In 421 B.C.E. Aristophanes wrote in his play, *Peace*, about the consequences of pennyroyal. In the play, Trigaius, who was about to mate with Harvesthome, lamented to the god Hermes that Harvesthome might become pregnant. "Not if you add a dose of pennyroyal," Hermes replied.[47] But by the time of Trotula, late in the Middle Ages, pennyroyal was listed as an emmenagogue, not an abortifacient.[48] The knowledge of pennyroyal as a birth control agent was not entirely lost by then. Just the same, among the illustrations in Pseudo-Apuleius's *Herbal*, drawn during the thirteenth century and now Vienna, Österreichische National-bibliothek MS lat. 93, there is a drawing of pennyroyal. In the lower right margin there is a young man holding a sprig of pennyroyal in one hand while his other operates a mortar and pestle. Looking on is a young lady reclining at an angle on a couch with one hand on her womb and with her legs demurely crossed. This picture is not necessarily an indication of birth control. However, I suggest that the ambiguity is there. Were pennyroyal merely intended as a menstrual regulator as the text of Pseudo-Apuleius indicated, would the artist have drawn the picture as he or she did?

As a generalization, the medieval church condemned abortion, but abortion generally was defined as termination of pregnancy after the fetus had formed. Prior to what commonly will be called in English quickening, there was a window or time period when the decision belonged to the woman.[49]

Why then are explicit references to birth control agents found increasingly less frequently in the medieval manuscripts and later in the printed books? Answers are complex, but I shall suggest a few. First, there was the organization of medicine with male university-trained physicians increasingly becoming the only legal practitioners. Medical education did not treat much gynecology and hardly any obstetrics. Second, the medieval church increased its strong stance against any form of birth control, including contraception and even fertility enhancers. Third, the period from approximately 1000 to 1300 was one of rapid population growth and even a pronatal movement, we suppose, among the common folk. The trail of learning about birth control nearly broke off completely and, as a widespread practice, its effect was negligible.

In the nineteenth century, in many countries including the United States, abortion was made a criminal offense. In 1869, Pope Pius IX declared that life began at conception. The medical profession did not strongly resist the new Catholic position because the time of quickening was a woman's determination. Yet, physicians were criminally responsible for the termination of any pregnancy. In 1848, the American physician Charles Meigs said, "The stupidest thing a physician can do, is to be misled by complaints to administering drugs and medicines, which may bring on, not the menses, but an abortion, or premature labor."[50]

How do we know that medieval women took emmenagogues as birth control agents? The evidence from the manuscripts mentioned here indicates that at least some people were aware of such agents. We also infer that they took or did something because we know that the family sizes were less than would be indicated by assuming that normal biological urges to mate were gratified on a regular basis.

## NOTES

1. Pliny, *Natural History*, W.H.S. Jones, H. Rackham, and D.E. Eicholz, eds. and trans., 10 vols. (Cambridge, MA: Harvard University Press, 1929–1971) 20. 51. 143; Galen, *De antidotis*, 2. 1 (*Claudii Galeni Opera omnia*, Karl Gottlob Kühn, ed., 22 vols. [Hildesheim: Olms, 1821–1833, repr. 1964–65] 14: 109–111).

2. Soranus, *Gynaecology*, Oswei Temkin, ed. and trans. (Baltimore: Johns Hopkins University Press, 1956) 1. 63. For the Greek text, see *Sorani Gynaeciorum libri IV*, Johannes Ilberg, ed., *Corpus Medicorum Graecorum* 4 (Leipzig and Berlin: Teubner, 1927) 47.

3. For discussion of rue, see Dioscorides, *De materia medica*, Max Wellmann, ed., 3 vols. (Berlin: Weidmann, 1958) 3. 45.

4. Added to margin in another hand in Vienna MS med. gr. 16, s. xv, and several other manuscripts including Vatican Palat. MS 77, s. xiv, and printed in the critical apparatus to Dioscorides, *De materia medica*, 3. 45 (Wellmann ed., 2: 59).

5. John Thomas Noonan, Jr., *Contraception: A History of Its Treatment by the Catholic Theologians and Canonists*, rev. ed. (Cambridge, MA: Harvard University Press, 1986).

6. Josiah Cox Russell, *The Control of Late Ancient and Medieval Population* (Philadelphia: American Philosophical Society, 1985).

7. David Herlihy, *Medieval Households* (Cambridge, MA: Harvard University Press, 1985) 146–149.

8. George A. Conway and John C. Slocumb, "Plants Used as Abortifacients and Emmenagogues by Spanish New Mexicans," *Journal of Ethnopharmacology* 1 (1979): 247–248; Martha O. Guerra and Amaury T.L. Andrade, "Contraceptive Effects of Native Plants in Rats," *Contraception* 18 (1978): 191–199, esp. 198; James A. Duke, *CRC Handbook of Medicinal Herbs* (Boca Raton, FL: CRC Press, 1985) 417; B.S. Malhi and V.P. Trivedi, "Vegetable Antifertility Drugs of India," *Quarterly Journal of Crude Drug Research* 12 (1972): 1927.

9. Yun Cheung Kong, C.P. Lau, K.H. Wat, K.H. Ng, P.H. But, K.F. Cheng, and P.G. Waterman, "Antifertility Principle of Ruta graveolens," *Planta Medica* 55 (1989): 1–44.

10. Yun Cheung Kong, K.H. Ng, K.H. Wat, A. Wong, I.F. Saxena, F.F. Cheng, P.H. But, and H.T. Chang, "Yuehchukene, a Novel Anti-implantation Indole Alkaloid from *Murraya paniculata*," *Planta Medica* 51 (1985): 304–307.

11. *The Merck's Index,* P.G. Stecher, ed., 7th ed. (Rahway, NJ: Merck, 1960) 818.

12. Pliny, *Natural History,* 20. 51. 139.

13. Johannes Fischer, *Die Gynäkologie bei Dioskurides und Plinius* (Vienna: Julius Springer, 1927) 6–7.

14. Pliny, *Natural History,* 20. 51. 143.

15. Philadelphia, College of Physicians, MS 10. a. 159, fol. 39ra.

16. Gargilius Martialis, *Medicinae ex oleribus et pomis* 3, ed.Valentin Rose, (Leipzig: Teubner, 1875) 137; trans. Ruth M. Tapper, diss. University of Wisconsin, 1980, 26).

17. Dioscorides, *De materia medica* 1. 81 (Wellmann ed., 1. 79).

18. Munich MS lat. 337, H. Mihàescu, ed. (Iasi, Romania: Alexander Terek, 1938) 48.

19. Dioscorides, *De materia medica* 1. 81 (Wellmann ed., 1, 79).

20. Munich MS lat. 337, H. Mihàescu, ed., 48.

21. Dioscorides, *De materia medica* 2. 159 (3. 4–5; Wellmann ed., 1, 225): ἄγει καὶ ἔμβρυα. ἀτόκιον δὲ εἶναι δοκεῖ μετὰ συνουσίαν προστιθέμενον.

22. [Anony. Latin], *De materia medica* 2. PME (Hermann Stadler, ed. *Romanische Forschungen* 10 [1897] 233).

23. Dioscorides, *De materia medica* 2. 156 (2. 4; Wellmann ed., 1, 223); Stadler, 10, 232; cf. virtually the same in Anony. Latin, *De mat. med.* 2. PLGP (Stadler, 10, 432).

24. Oribasius, *Ecologae medicamentorum* 632, *Oribasii collectionum medicarum reliuquiae,* Johannes Raeder, ed., 5 vols. (Leipzig and Berlin: Teubner, 1928–1933, repr. Amsterdam, 1964) 6, pt. 2, fasc. 2, p. 302.

25. Oribasius, *Synopsis, Oribasius Latinus,* Henning Mørland, ed. (Oslo: A.W. Brøgger, 1940) 75, 118, 148.

26. John M. Riddle, *Contraception and Abortion from the Ancient World to the Renaissance* (Cambridge, MA: Harvard University Press, 1992).

27. (Pseudo-Dioscorides), *Ex herbis feminis,* no. 28, Heinrich Kästner, ed., *Hermes* 31: 595): "sucus earum cum lana genitalibus iniectus abortionem praegnantibus facit."

28. R.R. Chaudhury, "Plants with Possible Antifertility Activity," *Indian Council for Medical Research: Special Reports Series* 55 (1966): 11 [1–19]; L. Palma, *Le piante medicinali d'Italia: botanica, chimica,*

*farmacodinamica, terapia* (Rome: Societá Editrice Internazionale, 1964) 563.

29. Oribasius, *Synopsis* 2 (Mørland ed., 148): *"artemisia trita et puleiu et centauria et thimu et ruta et alia omnia qui tali sunt virtute."*

30. Oribasius, *Synopsis* (Mørland ed., 75, 118, 148).

31. *Herbarium Apulei*, no. 158, ed. Thomas Oswald Cockayne, *Leechdoms, Wortcunning and Starcraft of Early England*, 3 vols., 1864, Repr. London: Kraus, 1965) 1: 312.

32. B.B. Sharma, M.D. Varshney, D.N. Gupta, and A.O. Prakash, "Antifertility Screening of Plants. Part I: Effect of Ten Indigenous Plants on Early Pregnancy in Albino Rats," *International Journal of Crude Drug Research* 21 (1983): 185; James A. Duke, *CRC Handbook of Medicinal Herbs* (Boca Raton, FL: CRC Press, 1985) 502.

33. I am relying on the *Patrologiae* edition. I have not seen the newly identified manuscripts of Hildegard that are found in Vatican, MS Ferraioli 921 and Florence, MS Laur. Ashb. 1323. Reading of these texts may shed more light on the alleged emendation.

34. Hildegard, *Physica*, no. 111 (*PL* 197:1174).

35. Duke, 474; *Tabers Cyclopedic Medical Dictionary*, 6th ed., (Philadelphia: Davis, 1954), s.v. ecbolic.

36. Hildegard, *Physica*, no. 42 (*PL* 198: 1148).

37. Hildegard, *Physica*, no. 116 (*PL* 197: 1177).

38. Hildegard, *Physica*, no. 34 (*PL* 197: 1143): "Sed et pregnantem mulierum cum periculo corporis sui abortire facit, si eum comederit."

39. Peter of Padua, Gloss, printed in Latin Alphabetical Dioscorides (Colle: Per Johannem Allemanumde Medemblick, 1478), s.v. *Asarus:* "alia viridis herba ab asaros iam tacto quem autem sit ante coitum videtur ignorari."

40. Henry de Laszlo and Paul S. Henshaw, "Plants Used by Primitive Peoples to Affect Fertility," *Science* 119 (1954): 627; V.J. Brøndegaard, "Contraceptive Plant Drugs," *Planta Medica* 23 (1972): 168.

41. Soranus, *Gynaecology*, 1. 64; Dioscorides, *De materia medica*, 3. 113.

42. Pliny, *Natural History*, 20. 90. 151, 159; Oribasius, *Synopsis* 2 (Mørland ed., 148).

43. *Magic and Medicine of Plants* (Reader's Digest, 1986) 348.

44. Duke, *CRC Handbook*, 68–70; John M. Riddle and J. Worth Estes, *American Scientist* 80 (1992): 231.

45. Macer, *Aemilius Macer De herbarum virtutibus. . . .* Apud Friburgum Brisgoicum, 1530, fol. 1: "Pellit abortuum potu, vel subdita tantum."

46. Macer, fol. 38.

47. Aristophanes, *Peace,* in *Knights, Lysistrata, Peace,* 3 vols., ed. and trans. Benjamin Bickley Rogers, (Cambridge, MA: Harvard University Press, 1946–1950) 2: 64–65.

48. Trotula, [*Gynaecology*] in *Gynaeciorum hoc est De mulierum tum aliis,* eds. Conrad Gesner and Caspar Wolf, (Basel: Thomas Guarinus, 1566), cols. 222–223.

49. The evidence is more completely given in my *Contraception and Abortion from the Ancient World to the Renaissance* (Cambridge, MA: Harvard University Press, 1992). I am currently working on a sequel to cover the modern period.

50. Charles D. Meigs, *Females and Their Diseases* (Philadelphia: Lea and Blanchard, 1848) 405.

# The Medical Manuscripts of the Bibliotheca Palatina

*Debra L. Stoudt*

In the course of the Middle Ages the study of medicine underwent numerous dramatic changes. Medicine of the High Middle Ages still reflected classical traditions, and medical literature and practices of the period were primarily an amalgam of Greek, Latin, and Arabic scientific knowledge. The type of medicine taught at medieval universities was essentially Galenic, based as it was upon the works of this Greek authority.[1] With the Renaissance came a revival of interest in classical medicine, but also discoveries in the areas of anatomy, pathology, and physiology, which cast doubts on some traditional medical doctrines. In sixteenth-century Germany, Theophrastus Bombastus von Hohenheim (1493–1541), called Paracelsus, kindled interest in yet another facet of medicine with his rejection of a Humanistic approach in favor of alchemical remedies. The division between Galenic and Paracelsian medicine in sixteenth-century Germany reveals the ambiguous relationship between medicine, magic, and religion that, in fact, had existed for centuries throughout Europe. Despite advances in medical knowledge in the late Middle Ages, there remains a discrepancy between theory and practice, between medieval tradition, influenced by folk medicine closely associated with Christian practices and beliefs, and Renaissance innovation. Nowhere is the discrepancy more apparent than in the medical manuscripts found in the Bibliotheca Palatina.

The Bibliotheca Palatina refers to the collection of the electoral princes of the Palatinate, the *Kurfürsten* who resided in Heidelberg. The library included volumes that they and others donated to the curatorship of Heidelberg University, as well as the personal collection of the Palatine electors.

This chapter undertakes a brief history of the Bibliotheca Palatina, which is inextricably intertwined with the growth of Heidelberg University and the fortunes of the Palatine electors. Following is a characterization of the content of the medical manuscripts and an examination of how and why the Bibliotheca Palatina came to possess such impressive and diverse medical holdings. The statutes of the medical faculty of the university influenced the type and quantity of medical literature acquired for the Bibliotheca Palatina, but the personal interests of the Palatine electors had an even more profound impact on the library's development.

With the Golden Bull of 1356, Karl IV officially bestowed upon the *Kurfürsten* their special privileges, and since the electorate was an inherited position among the secular princes, the houses thus designated became political axes and their residences intellectual and cultural centers.[2] The eastern expansion of the twelfth and thirteenth centuries and the rise of the Habsburg and Bohemian dynasties had led to the founding of the first German university, the university in Prague, in 1348. Ruprecht I, the first Palatine elector (1353–1390), was eager to establish a center of learning in the western part of the Holy Roman Empire, and in 1386, he authorized the creation of a university in Heidelberg.[3]

Heidelberg University, like its prototype in Paris, consisted of four faculties: the *untere Fakultät* (the arts faculty or *Artistenfakultät*, which became known as the *philosophische Fakultät* by the sixteenth century); and the three *obere Fakultäten*: theology, law, and medicine. The upper and lower faculties each had their own library but there was some overlapping with regard to the holdings. Whereas the library of the upper faculties contained only works specific to the three disciplines, the arts library possessed not only works seminal to the study of the *artes liberales* but also some volumes dealing with the higher disciplines.

The libraries were created and augmented primarily through contributions from two sources: the professors and the electors. The tradition of bequests by professors and masters began with the first administrators of the university, whose contributions were also the most substantial ones during the early years.[4] In 1390, the first chancellor of the university, Konrad von Gelnhausen, bequeathed to the arts faculty library some two hundred manuscripts, most of a theological or juridical nature.[5] Six years later the university library inherited approximately 250 manuscripts belonging to the first rector, Marsilius of Inghen, who served in that capacity nine times during the first seven years of the university's existence.[6] Although Marsilius was a professor of the arts faculty, his personal library included several medical volumes, among which were works by Rhazes and Galen, the *Antidotarium Nicolai*, and the dietetic and uroscopic work of Isaac Judaeus.[7]

The other source of volumes for the Bibliotheca Palatina was the electors themselves. Ruprecht I, the founder of the university, contributed to the university's collection, as did his nephew, Ruprecht II, who donated manuscripts confiscated from the Jews who were driven from Heidelberg in 1390.[8] However, it was Ludwig III (*Kurfürst* 1410–1436), the great-grandnephew of the first elector, whose bequest most greatly enhanced the university libraries' holdings during the first fifty years.

In 1421 Ludwig bequeathed his personal book collection, until then housed in the Heidelberg castle, to the recently established library in the Heiliggeistkirche. Ludwig's father, Ruprecht III, had initiated construction of the church around 1400, but Ludwig directed that the galleries be designed to accommodate the books. Since 1413 the university had supervised the library in the Heiliggeistkirche; in that year the university appointed its professors to the twelve prebends of the cathedral church, thereby securing the relationship between the two institutions. When Ludwig's will was executed in 1438, two years after his death, some 162 volumes—89 theological, 12 juridical, 55 medical, and 6 astronomical/astrological texts—were relocated to the church.[9] The elector had stated that the works were intended for the use of professors, masters, and students; however, the restricted borrowing hours and the fact that the Heiliggeistkirche library was a *bibliotheca concatena,* that is, a library in which the codices were chained to large desks, greatly inhibited use.

Thus, by the first quarter of the fifteenth century, Heidelberg University laid claim to three libraries, two housed in the university library building, and the third in the Heiliggeistkirche. In 1466 a register of the volumes in the Bibliotheca Palatina (Heid. Hs. 47) was prepared according to the location of the works. The list included the approximately three hundred books of the three upper faculties in the upper chamber of the library building and the 286 codices of the arts faculty in the lower chamber on the ground floor. Some 134 volumes were housed in the library in the Heiliggeistkirche; by subject matter these included eighty theological, eleven juridical, thirty-two medical, and eleven liberal arts volumes.[10]

During the reigns of Ludwig III's two sons, Ludwig IV (1436–1449) and Friedrich der Siegreiche (Frederick the Victorious, regent 1449–1452; *Kurfürst* 1452–1476), the renown of the university declined due to bickering among the faculty and confrontations between the students and the townspeople. However, when Ludwig IV's son Philipp der Aufrichtige (Philip the Upright) became elector in 1476, he fostered his personal interest in books and learning by establishing at his court a circle of Humanist teachers and scholars whose influence eventually affected the university. This circle included Rudolf Agricola, Johann von Dalberg, Conrad Celtes, and Johann Reuchlin.[11] In this intellectual atmosphere Philipp reared his sons. Ludwig V, successor to the electorate (1508–1544), was known as the "Peacemaker" (der Friedfertige) and was intent on maintaining peace as the Reformation swept through Germany;[12] however, his nephew and later successor, Otto Heinrich (*Kurfürst* 1556–1559), took a strong stand in support of the new religion. Ludwig V and Otto Heinrich were the most avid bibliophiles among the Palatine electors, despite the profound political concerns during their reigns and the brief tenure of the latter.

Beginning with Ludwig V, the *Kurfürsten* also demonstrated an increased interest in all facets of the healing arts, which accounts for the significant number of hippo-pathological, pharmacological, and alchemical manuscripts acquired for the

Bibliotheca Palatina during the sixteenth century and first quarter of the seventeenth century. The Palatine electors themselves contributed liberally to the development of the university libraries' collections and encouraged their friends to do likewise. One such benefactor was Ulrich Fugger, a friend of Otto Heinrich and an Augsburg patrician, who, persecuted for his religious beliefs in his native city, sought refuge in Heidelberg in 1567; Fugger bequeathed his manuscript and printed book collection to Kurfürst Friedrich IV.[13] Because the collection was not immediately and accurately inventoried, and because Fugger continued to augment his collection after settling in Heidelberg, it is not known how many volumes of Fugger provenance became part of the Bibliotheca Palatina with Ulrich's death in 1584; however, more than 23,500 pounds (235 *Zentner*) of books initially were transported from Augsburg to Heidelberg.[14] The collection boasted an abundance of medical manuscripts and printed volumes, since not only Fugger himself but also many of those who helped him acquire the works manifested great interest in the discipline. Achilles Pirmin Gasser was one such individual. A doctor and personal friend of the family, he procured books for his own collection and for that of the Fuggers; at his death in 1577, Gasser's library boasted some 2,900 titles, 907 of which pertained to medicine. Ulrich Fugger acquired the bulk of the collection after his friend's death.[15]

Although the electors bequeathed a number of volumes to the university, they also maintained a private library, which consisted of particularly valuable manuscripts and volumes the electors had commissioned for their personal use. This collection was housed in Heidelberg castle, but by the time of Ludwig V's reign, it had expanded to such an extent that the elector made plans to build a new library at the castle. The building process began during Otto Heinrich's electorate; in the interim the surplus volumes were stored in the Heiliggeistkirche. However, with Otto Heinrich's death in 1559, construction of the new castle library was abandoned.[16]

By the seventeenth century, there were four major library collections in Heidelberg that comprised the Bibliotheca Palatina;[17] the sum of their manuscripts and printed works was about 9,500![18] The Bibliotheca Palatina justifiably was accorded the epithet of "the mother of all libraries," not only because of the extensiveness of the holdings, but also because of their superior quality. In addition to Latin and vernacular volumes, there were collections of Greek and oriental manuscripts, the latter acquired primarily by Otto Heinrich during a trip to the East. The electors also procured manuscripts from monastic communities, often borrowing volumes and then never returning them. In 1552, Kurfürst Friedrich II proclaimed the secularization of monastic institutions in the Palatinate. His nephew Otto Heinrich, still Palatine count of Neuburg at the time, took advantage of the decree to carry off more than seventy manuscripts from the nearby community of Lorsch, among them the *Lorscher Evangeliar* (Cpl. Vat. 50).[19] Although the Bibliotheca Palatina acquired primarily theological works from Lorsch,[20] the scriptoria of religious communities often served as an important source of medical manuscripts. Before the establishment of universities in Europe in the eleventh and twelfth centuries, medical practice had been the exclusive prerogative of the clergy. Even after the Church attempted to curtail medical activities among the clergy by means of various council decrees in the twelfth and thirteenth centuries, clerics continued their study and practice of medicine. The holdings of the monastic libraries reflect the dual role of spiritual and physical healer that the community members continued to play throughout the Middle Ages.

In 1623, early in the Thirty Years' War, the Austrian commander Tilly conquered Heidelberg and the holdings of the Bibliotheca Palatina were carried off to Rome the following year.[21] Duke Maximilian I of Bavaria relinquished the collection to Pope Gregory XV, in part because of the latter's support of the duke in the conflict, but also in acquiescence to the Pope's great interest in the volumes. The Bibliotheca Palatina was incorporated into the Vatican Library, and although the German manuscripts as well as some others were returned to Heidelberg in the course of the nineteenth century, the majority of the Latin manuscripts are still in Rome today.[22]

Medical literature of the Middle Ages encompassed a wide variety of topics. The theoretical treatises focused on diagnosis—

primarily by means of monitoring the pulse and the inspection of urine—and on prognosis. Therapeutic recommendations took various forms: Great emphasis was placed on diet and on herbal and other remedies, which gave rise to dietetic regimens, pharmacopoeias, herbals, collections of magical remedies, and lapidaries. In addition, certain surgical procedures, particularly phlebotomy and cautery, played a prominent role in the literature. In the Middle Ages it was generally accepted that the planets influenced the four humors, all of which were contained in blood; this gave rise to the preparation of calendars that listed the *verworfene Tage* (unfavorable days), on which one was to avoid bloodletting.

The study of medicine was the exclusive privilege of the learned and was within the purview of the clergy until the founding of the universities; for this reason the early manuscripts were written in Latin. Beginning in the twelfth century, when the first centers for medical studies were established in Western Europe and different classifications of healers emerged, medical literature in the vernacular appeared.[23]

Among the manuscripts of the Bibliotheca Palatina were 170 German and 270 Latin medical manuscripts.[24] The collection represented the scope of medical studies in the Middle Ages and was one of the largest of its type in German-speaking Europe. The Bibliotheca Palatina became a repository for medical manuscripts because of cultural, political, and socioeconomic developments in the Palatinate in late medieval times; the academic standards of the medical faculty at the university, the personal interest and support of the Palatine electors, and the concern of both with the well-being of Heidelberg's inhabitants contributed to the attention accorded medical literature.

The medical faculty in Heidelberg was established already in 1387 or 1390, shortly after the founding of the university itself, but this upper faculty did not grow at the same rate or flourish as did the others.[25] Only in 1482 was a second "ordentlicher Lehrer für Medizin" approved, and a third was added in 1522, despite the fact that only fourteen medical students were enrolled in 1520.[26] The modest size of Heidelberg's medical faculty reflected the prevailing situation at German universities during the later Middle Ages; among the sixteen oldest universities in German-speaking areas, the medical faculty was always the smallest of the four faculties.[27] The size of the medical faculty and the at times meager number of students at Heidelberg University could have inhibited the expansion of medical resources, but the high caliber and professional activity of the medical faculty, as well as the personal interest of the electors, preserved the integrity of the study of medicine.

The oldest manuscripts of the Heidelberg medical collection contain the traditional medieval medical works. In 1425 the medical faculty introduced statutes based on those adopted by the University of Cologne some thirty years earlier (1393). According to the statutes, the bachelors, that is, holders of the baccalaureate, had a reading list that was to be mastered before they became licentiates.[28] The works included in the list are those of the *Articella*, the collection of medical translations that served as the basis for medical study beginning in the twelfth century. Not surprisingly, the earliest bequests to the university libraries reflect the importance accorded the works of the classical and Arabic masters. Although the inventory of manuscripts bequeathed by Konrad von Gelnhausen contains none of the works cited in the statutes, the list of works donated by Marsilius of Inghen includes the names of Galen and Rhazes. Among the fifty-five medical volumes Ludwig III contributed to the Heiliggeistkirche library in 1421, one finds a majority of the works of the *Articella*. The numerous manuscripts of tracts by Galen, Rhazes, and Avicenna bespeak the emphasis placed on traditional authorities. However, the works of more contemporary European teachers, for example, Albertus Magnus, Arnold of Villanova, and those by local masters, such as Conradus de Eichstätt and Burkhard von Waltdorf-Wolfferen also are included; from Ludwig the library acquired a one-volume copy of Hildegard of Bingen's *Causae et curae* as well.[29]

The mixture of traditional and contemporary medical knowledge is also reflected in the manuscript contributions of the medical faculty. The electors' personal physicians, who usually were university professors, were men of renown actively engaged in the collection and transcription of medical literature. They fostered the tradition of manuscript bequests within their own faculty by contributing volumes they had purchased, copied, or drafted themselves during their tenure in Heidelberg. According to the inventory of the manuscripts bequeathed by Ludwig III, five of the volumes that contained medical tracts were written at least in part by Burkhard von Waltdorf-Wolfferen, personal physician of Ruprecht I and Ruprecht III and vice-chancellor of the university under Konrad von Gelnhausen.[30] Other significant contributors among the Heidelberg professors of medicine included Gerhard von Hohenkirchen (+1448), Heinrich Münsinger (ca. 1397–ca. 1476), Erhard Knab (+1480), Martinus Rentz (1480–1503), Konrad Schelling (+1514), and Johann Pleniger-Egen (+1544?).[31] The particularly noteworthy accomplishments of several of these men will be mentioned below in the discussion of the electors' personal interests.

Already in the twelfth and thirteenth centuries a tradition of medical literature in the vernacular had begun to emerge in Western Europe. By the end of the thirteenth century this development was flourishing in German-speaking areas as scribes copied and disseminated versions of works such as Ortolf von Baierland's *Arzneibuch*, the *Cirurgia* of Peter von Ulm, and the *Ordnung der Gesundheit*.[32] With the innovation in language, there was a concomitant shift in the intended audience. Whereas the Latin works clearly were intended for university-trained men of medicine, the vernacular works could be of use to village doctors (*badaere*), barber-surgeons (*bartscheraere*), and lay physicians.[33]

This dichotomy is one reason for the large number of Latin as well as German medical manuscripts in the Bibliotheca Palatina. Whereas the Latin manuscripts are primarily those written or acquired by university professors in the fourteenth and fifteenth centuries, most of the German medical manuscripts in the collection date from the fifteenth and sixteenth centuries and were purchases and autographs by the Palatine electors. Ludwig III's bequest to the university consisted solely of Latin manuscripts, because the university had no need of works in the vernacular; however, references in the texts themselves offer evidence that Ludwig possessed manuscripts in German, at least one of which dealt with hippopathology and human medicine.[34]

A majority of both the Latin and the German medical manuscripts in the Bibliotheca Palatina are *Sammelbände* or *Sammelhandschriften*. Often the authoritative sources were rather brief or had been excerpted from the oeuvre of the medical master; the individual tracts were then collected and bound in a single volume. Because many of the works were employed as university texts, the masters frequently added glosses and commentary in the margins. Since the tracts often were bound together at a later time, extraneous material was appended between the major portions of text or to the beginning or end of a collection of medical works. Such additions commonly took the form of remedies, because of the brevity of the recipes.[35]

The university designated funds every year for the purchase of books, but in the fifteenth and sixteenth centuries other types of medical volumes—some might say pseudomedical works—were acquired for the Bibliotheca Palatina at a more rapid rate. These included hippopathological works, folkloric cures and incantations, and works devoted to astrological medicine and alchemy. Each of these trends in manuscript and book collecting can be traced to the interests and personal health of the Palatine electors.

Like many of the nobility, the electors were avid hunters. Ludwig III seemed to have been particularly interested in falconry. It was he who probably commissioned two works on the subject: the *Buch von haltung, krankheiten und arzneien der falken, hunde und pferde*, Cpg. 206, translated by Werner Ernesti, professor of canon law in 1404;[36] and the *Buch von den falcken, habichen, sperbern, pferden vnd hůnden*, Cpg. 281, prepared by Ludwig's personal physician Heinrich Münsinger around 1440.[37] Both were translations of portions of the *De animalibus* of Albertus Magnus. In the seventeenth century the Bibliotheca Palatina acquired additional works on natural history through the endeavors of the Palatine regent and administrator Johann Casimir, a hunter par excellence who represented the "Jäger aus Kurpfalz" immortalized in folksong. Under Friedrich IV and Friedrich V, a copy of Kaiser Friedrich II's book of falconry was added to the library's holdings during the first quarter of the seventeenth century.[38]

An important part of literature on veterinary medicine was the specialized works dealing with the care and curing of horses, the *Roßarzneibücher*. The royal stables, erected on the banks of the Neckar, still stand today as a monument not only to the political authority of the electors but also to their fondness of horses. There are more than three dozen manuscripts containing hippopathological material, two-thirds of which are written in the vernacular. These manuscripts contain tracts describing various illnesses as well as remedies, some copied and even tested by the electors themselves.[39] The son of Philipp der Aufrichtige—also named Philipp—Palatine count and Bishop of Freising, compiled his own *Roßarzneibuch* around 1500. His brother, Ludwig V, successor to the electorate, himself copied some 450 pages of hippopathological recipes and tracts from various sources (Cpg. 255).[40]

The electors were concerned with the well-being of their horses, but more importantly with their own health. Particularly in their later years, a number of the electors suffered from various maladies and often commissioned their personal physicians to collect remedies or prepare dietetic regimens for their personal use. Friedrich I, who suffered from a bronchial inflammation, commissioned Heinrich Münsinger to prepare a vernacular version of his *Regimen sanitatis in fluxu catarrhali ad pectus*.[41] Friedrich also authorized Erhard Knab to provide him with a pharmacopoeia.[42] Ludwig V did his own collecting and claimed to have applied some of the medical cures himself.[43] Otto Heinrich also compiled remedies. Some addressed the effectiveness of mineral springs (*Regement zu gebrauchen das wildbad*, Cpg. 683, f. 18r), of which the elector partook on a regular basis;[44] others dealt with health precautions to follow while traveling (*Wie man sich in der kellte zu raisen oder zureitten halten soll*, Cpg. 683, f. 30v). Ludwig VI, sickly from youth, had a *Diätbuch* prepared for his personal use.[45]

The examples just cited offer evidence of the personal interest of several electors in medical matters, an interest so great that the electors themselves copied the material. The most impressive of these undertakings was carried out by Ludwig V between 1526 and his death in 1544. Ludwig copied some three thousand pages of medical knowledge, recipes, and incantations from manuscripts borrowed and purchased from local practitioners of medicine and physicians at neighboring courts; the result of this arduous activity was the *Zwölfbändiges Buch der Medizin*, Cpg. 261–272, which was bound and dedicated to Ludwig's memory in 1554, ten years after his death.

The *Zwölfbändiges Buch der Medizin* is the Palatine electors' greatest monument to medical knowledge and best exemplifies the ambiguous political position of the Palatinate and the analogous position of Heidelberg University, caught between languishing Scholastic thought and the nascent Renaissance and Humanist tendencies. Ludwig's volumes include excerpts from vernacular versions of tracts by classical and Arabic medical authors, for example, Hippocrates, Galen, Avicenna, Rhazes, and Johannitius, as well as passages from the more contemporary German sources mentioned above, for example, Ortolf von Baierland, Peter von Ulm, and the *Ordnung der Gesundheit*. Interspersed among the tracts are herbal recipes that resemble those found in Dioscorides and the *Circa instans*, two standard sources. In addition there are medical-astrological cures and approximately four hundred incantations and charms among the twenty thousand entries. Although the percentage of magical cures is modest, their inclusion in Ludwig's volumes is most noteworthy.[46] Whereas incantations often were relegated to the margins and fly leaves of medieval manuscripts, Ludwig copied them alongside herbal and other remedies, an indication that in sixteenth-century Heidelberg there was evidently a strong belief in, or at least curiosity surrounding the use of charms for healing purposes.

The digression from traditional medical teachings intensified under Otto Heinrich, who despite his brief tenure as elector (1556–1559), profoundly affected the politico-religious and educational environment in the Palatinate. Otto Heinrich was a devotee of academic pursuits and dedicated a substantial portion of his resources to the acquisition of new volumes. Like many people in his day, the elector believed in astrology and collected many books on the subject for his personal library. Interest in astrology and the occult, particularly as they pertained to medicine, had been rekindled by the works of Paracelsus and his followers; their doctrines dramatically influenced medical teaching and practice for the next century, although very few of the Swiss alchemist's works were published during his lifetime.[47] Even before Paracelsus's death in 1541, Hans Kilian, a chemist and confidant of Otto Heinrich, arranged for the acquisition of an impressive collection of autographs and other Paracelsian manuscripts for the personal library of the future elector, at the time still the Palatine count of Neuburg.[48] Several years later, Otto Heinrich brought the manuscripts to the attention of his personal physician Alexander von Suchten; recognizing the contentious nature of Paracelsian remedies, Otto Heinrich ordered that his physician not publish any of the manuscript material without his knowledge, but Suchten was permitted to test the cures.[49] Other men of medicine in Otto Heinrich's service—Michael Schütz (Toxites), Wilhelm Rascalon, and Adam von Bodenstein—also devoted years of study to the alchemical manuscripts; most of their own works on the subject appeared in the two decades following the elector's death. Otto Heinrich's interest in alchemy is reflected in his substantial collection of manuscripts and printed texts on the subject, in addition to the Paracelsian manuscripts. Among them are the alchemical tracts of Cpg. 467, a translation of the *Margaritha philosophorum* in Cpg. 801, and the two-part *Alchimia opuscula* (Stamp. Pal. IV 507 [lat. 916] and Stamp. Pal. IV 326).[50]

Aside from natural curiosity about alchemical medicine, there may have been other reasons for Otto Heinrich's interest in the occult. In a recent study of patronage at German courts during the early modern period, Bruce T. Moran states that projects supported by the princes often were tied to the political or economic ambitions of the patron.[51] Particularly at Protestant German courts, princes turned to alchemy and the occult "as an act of political desperation."[52] In an attempt to counterbalance the Catholic views of the Habsburg empire, the Protestant princes attempted to forge their own court philosophy based on science and the occult arts. Otto Heinrich's political circumstances were not as dire as those of the princes of the subsequent century, but his extravagant lifestyle beset him with health and financial problems. The elector's interest in Paracelsus's writings probably centered upon the "Lapis philosophorum," which was thought to restore good health, and the alchemical application of

Paracelsus's ideas, that is, the transmutation of base metals into gold.[53] Otto Heinrich's circumspect support of Paracelsian medical philosophy portended the overt patronage that German courts of the seventeenth century would provide to the physicians who followed the *medicina hermetica*.[54]

It is perhaps ironic that during this time the revision of the statutes of the medical faculty should have been accepted. The reforms had been recommended by Johann Lange, the personal physician of Friedrich II, Otto Heinrich's predecessor. Although Lange's ideas about medical practice were in some ways progressive, letters by the doctor offer proof that he held to beliefs in the humors and in exorcism.[55] Nonetheless, Lange is numbered among the Heidelberg Humanist doctors of the sixteenth century, a list which also includes Thomas Erastus, the great opponent of Paracelsus, and Johann Virdung. It was during the reign of Friedrich III, Otto Heinrich's successor, that Erastus was active at the university as a staunch adherent of the traditional Galenic school of medicine and defender of the *medicina dogmatica* against the *medicina hermetica* of Paracelsus.[56] In part because of his theological beliefs, Erastus took issue with Paracelsus's concept of natural magic;[57] likewise, he would not condone Paracelsus's acceptance of, or at least ambivalence toward the occult arts. Johann Virdung of Haßfurth, a doctor of medicine, taught astronomy and medicine and was also court mathematician under Philipp and Ludwig V; in addition he held the position of court apothecary. Famous for his astronomical tables, Virdung was also interested in magic and was said to have been visited by Georgus Faustus in 1507.[58]

The acquisition of medical literature for the Bibliotheca Palatina was an academic as well as a bibliophilistic pursuit, but the collection also reflects a concern with the practical application of medical knowledge to benefit the common man. The electors commissioned dietetic regimens and personally copied recipes for cures to their own afflictions, but there was a larger body of medical literature that focused on more widespread medical problems, for example, plague and leprosy.

The Black Death swept through Europe repeatedly in the late Middle Ages. The annual flooding of the Neckar, which submerged much of the old part of the city, made Heidelberg particularly susceptible to the ravages of this pestilence.[59] The epidemic in 1491 was so devastating that Philipp der Aufrichtige fled the city, and the university was relocated temporarily to Speyer. Between 1426 and 1597, the university community deserted the city nineteen times.[60] In the Bibliotheca Palatina there are more than seventy-five manuscripts containing tracts describing the plague and remedies against it. The tracts, primarily in Latin, are of foreign origin, for example, Pietro da Tussignano (Cpl. 1260, 121ra–172ra) and Marsilio Ficino (Cpl. 1338, 45r). The source of the recipes, more than half of which are in the vernacular, is often omitted. Heidelberg masters such as Erhard Knab, Thomas Erastus, and Konrad Schelling showed particularly keen interest in literature on the plague.[61]

The literature on leprosy in the Heidelberg collection is less extensive. All of the tracts are contained in *Sammelhandschriften* and most are in Latin. Cpl. 1207, 147v–148v, contains reports by Gerhard von Hohenkirchen of examinations performed on people suspected of being infected with leprosy.[62] In Cpl. 1225, 16v, and Cpl. 1316, 101r, one finds remedies for the disease that Erhard Knab recorded or had recorded for his use.

The medical collection of the Bibliotheca Palatina, and indeed the library itself, were the product of both the intellectual concerns of the university professors and the personal interests of the Rhenish Wittelsbach rulers. In the fourteenth and fifteenth centuries, the scope of the medical works in the Bibliotheca Palatina reflected the state of the study of medicine in the High and Late Middle Ages. Among the medical manuscripts, one finds the works of Hippocrates and Galen; the Arabic tradition exemplified by Rhazes and Avicenna; the Scholastic contribution by the masters in Salerno, Paris, and Montpellier; and the local influence of the professors at the university in Heidelberg.

The rediscovery of Greek texts and the establishment of Heidelberg as a Humanist center at the end of the fifteenth century provided the impetus for the innovations, for example, the study of anatomy and pathology, and the reforms, such as the regulation of the licensing of physicians, within the medical faculty in the sixteenth century. The renewed emphasis on learning also may be perceived as the source of the alternate path of medical inquiry followed in sixteenth-century Heidelberg, particularly by the electors. At the same time the reforms were being implemented at the university, Ludwig V was focusing his attention on the collecting and recording of incantations and magic charms alongside traditional medical tracts, and Otto Heinrich was encouraging the acquisition and study of astrological and alchemical treatises, which led to a rift between the Galenic and Paracelsian camps within the medical faculty.

The divergent nature of the medical acquisitions for the Bibliotheca Palatina in the sixteenth century reflect the abandonment of the complete and indiscriminate acceptance of classical authorities and traditional remedies by those with medical training, as well as by the general public. The seemingly contradictory beliefs of a professor and doctor like Johann Lange and a layperson like Ludwig V—both of whom gave credence to scientific and nonscientific cures—offer evidence of the ambivalent attitude toward medicine prevalent among the learned and the laity in Heidelberg at the beginning of the modern age.

## NOTES

1. Nancy G. Siraisi's recent book, *Medieval and Early Renaissance Medicine. An Introduction to Knowledge and Practice* (Chicago and London: University of Chicago Press, 1990), offers an excellent general presentation of medicine in the Middle Ages. See also John M. Riddle, "Theory and Practice in Medieval Medicine," *Viator. Medieval and Renaissance Studies* 5 (1974): 157–184.

2. Elmar Mittler offers a concise explanation of the rights and privileges of the electoral princes, particularly the Palatine electors, in "Die Sonderstellung der Kurfürsten von der Pfalz im Heiligen Römischen Reich" in *Bibliotheca Palatina. Katalog zur Ausstellung vom 8. Juli bis 2. November 1986. Heiliggeistkirche Heidelberg. Textband*, ed. Elmar Mittler (Heidelberg: Universitätsbibliothek, 1986) 4–5. Henry J. Cohn characterizes the electors' political role in "The Golden Bull and the Family Treaties of the Electors Palatine" in *The Government of the Rhine Palatinate in the Fifteenth Century* (Oxford: Oxford University Press, 1965)

17–22. Martina Backes also undertakes an examination of the status of the Wittelsbach family and the significance of the Heidelberg court as a social and cultural center in *Das literarische Leben am kurpfälzischen Hof zu Heidelberg im 15. Jahrhundert. Ein Beitrag zur Gönnerforschung des Spätmittelalters*, Hermaea, n.s. 68 (Tübingen: Max Niemeyer, 1992) 7–44.

3. Ludwig Häusser chronicles the history of the Palatine electors in *Geschichte der Rheinischen Pfalz nach ihren politischen, kirchlichen und literarischen Verhältnissen*, 2 vols., 2nd ed. (1856; rpt. Pirmasens: Johann Richter, 1970). See also Meinrad Schaab, *Geschichte der Kurpfalz*, 2 vols. (Stuttgart: Kohlhammer, 1988 and 1992).

4. Gustav Toepke offers a list of the manuscripts bequeathed to the library between 1396 and 1432 in appendices III and IV of *Die Matrikel der Universität Heidelberg von 1386 bis 1662*. 1. Theil von 1386 bis 1553 (Heidelberg: Winter, 1884; rpt. Nendeln/Liechtenstein: Kraus, 1976) 655–695.

5. Reinhard Düchting, "Bibliotheca Palatina. Vom europäischen Glanz einer traditionsreichen Institution," *Heidelberger Jahrbücher* 29 (1985): 133.

6. Until 1393 elections for the position of rector were held four times a year. Hermann Weisert lists the university rectors and the deans of the individual faculties in "Die Rektoren und die Dekane der Ruperto Carola zu Heidelberg 1386–1985," *Semper apertus. Sechshundert Jahre Ruprecht-Karls-Universität Heidelberg 1386–1986. Festschrift in sechs Bänden*, ed. Wilhelm Doerr, Band IV: Übergreifende Beiträge (Berlin and Heidelberg: Springer, 1985) 299–407.

7. Marsilius's medical volumes are inventoried in Toepke, 681.

8. Toepke, 662.

9. Mittler, ed., *Bibliotheca Palatina*, 8.

10. Mittler, ed., *Bibliotheca Palatina*, 10–11.

11. Backes discusses the literary accomplishments of the Humanists in Philipp's court in *Das literarische Leben am kurpfälzischen Hof zu Heidelberg im 15. Jahrhundert*, 136–160.

12. Wolfgang Eger, "Kurfürst Ludwig V. der Friedfertige (von Wittelsbach), Pfalzgraf bei Rhein," in *Der Reichstag zu Worms von 1521. Reichspolitik und Luthersache*, ed. Fritz Reuter (Worms: Stadtarchiv Worms, 1971) 352–368.

13. Otto Heinrich had no heirs, nor did any of his siblings. Hence, with his death in 1559, the *alte Kurlinie* was extinguished and the Simmern line of the Rhenish Wittelsbachs assumed the electorate (the *mittlere Kurlinie*).

14. Paul Lehmann, *Eine Geschichte der alten Fuggerbibliothek. I. Teil*, Studien zur Fuggergeschichte 12 (Tübingen: J.C.B. Mohr [Paul Siebeck], 1956) 167–171. In the second volume of his study, *Eine Geschichte der alten Fuggerbibliothek. II. Teil*, Studien zur Fuggergeschichte 15, 1960, 472–550, Lehmann catalogues some 575 Latin and German Palatina manuscripts whose Fugger provenance is relatively certain. In his discussion of the Fugger library in *Bibliotheca Palatina*, 377, Elmar Mittler tallies five hundred parchment manuscripts, eight hundred paper manuscripts, and 8,200 printed works, citing, however, the same difficulties that Lehmann mentions in estimating the number of volumes from Fugger. See also Mittler's description of Fugger's library treasure in *Mit der Zeit. Die Kurfürsten von der Pfalz und die Heidelberger Handschriften der Bibliotheca Palatina*, Elmar Mittler and Wilfried Werner (Wiesbaden: Ludwig Reichert, 1986) 24–28.

15. Mittler, *Bibliotheca Palatina*, 399 and 413; the tabulation of titles according to topic is also found in Lehmann, *Eine Geschichte der alten Fuggerbibliothek. I. Teil*, 185.

16. Not all of Otto Heinrich's personal library was housed in the Heidelberg castle and the Heiliggeistkirche. Otto Heinrich was Palatine count of Neuburg from 1505 to 1556 and resided at his castle in Neuburg on the Donau during this time. At the age of fifty-four he finally assumed the Palatine electorate upon the death of his uncle Friedrich II and moved to Heidelberg, taking with him some but not all of his manuscript collection. Whereas Tilly's troops plundered the Heidelberg libraries at the beginning of the Thirty Years' War, the Neuburg collection was spared. Karl Schottenloher describes the fate of Otto Heinrich's personal library in *Pfalzgraf Ottheinrich und das Buch. Ein Beitrag zur Geschichte der evangelischen Publizistik. Mit Anhang: Das Reformationsschrifttum in der Palatina*, Reformationsgeschichtliche Studien und Texte 50/51 (Münster: Aschendorff, 1927) 3–39.

17. There were other smaller libraries in Heidelberg, e.g., the collection at the Dionysianum to which Gerhard von Hohenkirchen bequeathed his books.

18. Ludwig Schuba tallies the manuscripts that arrived at the Vatican Library according to language in *Die medizinischen Handschriften der Codices Palatini Latini in der Vatikanischen Bibliothek*, Kataloge der Universitätsbibliothek Heidelberg 1 (Wiesbaden: Reichert, 1981) X.

19. Schottenloher describes this incident in *Pfalzgraf Ottheinrich und das Buch*, 7–8.

20. See Bernhard Bischoff, *Lorsch im Spiegel seiner Handschriften*, Münchener Beiträge zur Mediävistik und Renaissance-Forschung, Beiheft (Munich: Arbeo-Gesellschaft, 1974) 96 and 104–119.

21. For a detailed account of this event, see Friedrich Wilken, *Geschichte der Bildung, Beraubung und Vernichtung der alten Heidelbergischen Büchersammlungen. Ein Beytrag zur Literaturgeschichte vornehmlich des 15. und 16. Jahrhunderts* (Heidelberg: Oswald, 1817); and Augustin Theiner, *Schenkung der Heidelberger Bibliothek durch Maximilian I., Herzog und Churfürsten von Bayern, an Papst Gregor XV. und ihre Versendung nach Rom* (Munich: Verlag der Lit. Art. Anstalt, 1844). Ludwig Hammermayer discusses the incorporation of the Heidelberg manuscripts into the collection in Rome in "Zur Geschichte der 'Bibliotheca Palatina' in der Vatikanischen Bibliothek. Briefe Johann Georg Loris aus Rom an Andreas Felix Öfele in München (1750/1751)," *Römische Quartalschrift für christliche Altertums kunde und Kirchengeschichte* 55 (1960): 1–41, and "Neue Beiträge zur Geschichte der Bibliotheca Palatina in Rom," *Römische Quartalschrift für christliche Altertumskunde und Kirchengeschichte* 57 (1962): 146–179.

22. Walter Berschin provides an imaginary tour of the Palatina in Rome and a description of some of its most notable manuscripts in *Die Palatina in der Vaticana. Eine deutsche Bibliothek in Rom* (Stuttgart: Belsen, 1992).

23. For more on medical literature in medieval Germany, see, e.g., Gerhard Eis, "Mittelalterliche Fachprosa der Artes," *Deutsche Philologie im Aufriß. Band II*, 2nd ed. (Berlin: Schmidt, 1960), cols. 1103–1216; Gerhard Eis, *Mittelalterliche Fachliteratur*, 2nd ed. (Stuttgart: Metzler, 1967); Gundolf Keil, "Die deutsche medizinische Literatur im Mittelalter" in *Verhandlungen des XX. Internationalen Kongresses für Geschichte der Medizin. Berlin, 22.-27. August 1966*, eds. Heinz Goerke and Heinz Müller-Dietz (Hildesheim: Georg Olms, 1968) 647–654; and Wolfgang Hirth, "Corpusbildung in der deutschsprachigen medizinischen Fachliteratur des Mittelalters," *Sudhoffs Archiv* 66 (1982): 239–275.

24. The following catalogues contain a description of the medical manuscripts in the Palatine collection: Karl Bartsch, *Die altdeutschen Handschriften der Universitäts-Bibliothek in Heidelberg*, Katalog der Handschriften der Universitäts-Bibliothek in Heidelberg, I (Heidelberg: Gustav Koester, 1887); Ludwig Schuba, *Die medizinischen Handschriften*; Jakob Wille, *Die deutschen Pfälzer Handschriften des XVI. und XVII. Jahrhunderts*, Katalog der Handschriften der Universitäts-Bibliothek in Heidelberg, II (Heidelberg: Gustav Koester, 1903).

25. The foundation and growth of the medical faculty at Heidelberg University during the period preceding the Thirty Years'

War is described in: Eberhard Stübler, *Geschichte der medizinischen Fakultät der Universität Heidelberg 1386–1925* (Heidelberg: Winter, 1926); Wilhelm Kühlmann and Joachim Telle, "Humanismus und Medizin an der Universität Heidelberg im 16. Jahrhundert," *Semper apertus*, Band I: Mittelalter und frühe Neuzeit 1386–1803, 255–289; and Heinrich Schipperges, "Ursprung und Schicksal der Medizinischen Fakultät," *Semper apertus*, Band IV, 49–91.

26. Stübler, 9. Stübler also notes that from the time of Ruprecht I, the electors retained the privilege of appointing the "ordentlicher Lehrer." Hence, it was not uncommon for the elector's personal physician to serve in the capacity of professor of medicine. As was the custom, all *doctores legentes* of medicine had to be clerics. It was only during the reign of Philipp der Aufrichtige (1476–1508) that the first layman was appointed to the position; the official installation of laymen in the position was granted in 1553. See Theodor Billroth, *Über das Lehren und Lernen der medicinischen Wissenschaften an den Universitäten der deutschen Nation nebst allgemeinen Bemerkungen über Universitäten* (Vienna: Carl Gerolds Sohn, 1876) 15.

27. Klaus Pielmeyer, *Statuten der deutschen medizinischen Fakultäten im Mittelalter*, diss. Bonn 1981 (Bonn: Richard Schwarzbold, 1981) 8.

28. Hermann Weisert, "Die ältesten Statuten der Medizinischen Fakultät Heidelbergs (1425)," *Ruperto-Carola* 33 (1981) 67.

29. For a complete list of the titles of the medical manuscripts donated by Ludwig III, see Schuba, *Die medizinischen Handschriften*, XXII–XXVII.

30. Schuba, *Die medizinischen Handschriften*, XXVII and XXVIII.

31. The following sources offer a detailed discussion of the accomplishments of these physicians and their manuscript contributions to the Bibliotheca Palatina: Ludwig Schuba, *Die medizinischen Handschriften*, XIX–XXXV; idem, "Die medizinische Fakultät im 15. Jahrhundert," *Semper apertus*, Band I, 164–168 and 171–182; and entries in *Die deutsche Literatur des Mittelalters. Verfasserlexikon*. Gerhard von Hohenkirchen, and probably Konrad Schelling as well, bequeathed their books to the Dionysianum, which, although evidently a separate collection, was supervised by the university (Schuba, *Die medizinischen Handschriften*, XXXI).

32. The content, sources, and transmission of these tracts are described in the critical editions: J[ames] Follan, *Das Arzneibuch Ortolfs von Baierland nach der ältesten Handschrift*, Veröffentlichungen der Internationalen Gesellschaft für Geschichte der Pharmazie 23 (Stuttgart: Wissenschaftliche Verlagsgesellschaft, 1963); Gundolf Keil, *Die 'Cirurgia'*

*Peters von Ulm. Untersuchungen zu einem Denkmal altdeutscher Fachprosa mit kritischer Ausgabe des Textes*, Forschungen zur Geschichte der Stadt Ulm 2 (Ulm: Stadtarchiv, 1961); Christa Hagenmeyer, "Die 'Ordnung der Gesundheit' für Rudolf von Hohenberg. Untersuchungen zur diätetischen Fachprosa des Spätmittelalters mit kritischer Textausgabe," diss. Heidelberg, 1972.

33. Gundolf Keil, "Ortolf von Baierland (von Würzburg), *Die deutsche Literatur des Mittelalters. Verfasserlexikon*, ed. Kurt Ruh, 2nd ed., vol. 7 (Berlin and New York: de Gruyter, 1987), col. 75.

34. The reference here is to Cpg. 206, the *Buch von haltung, krankheiten und arzneien der falken, hunde und pferde*, a description of which can be found in Bartsch, 47. Concerning Ludwig III's German manuscript collection, see Konrad Burdach, "Die pfälzischen Wittelsbacher und die altdeutschen Handschriften der Palatina," *Centralblatt für Bibliothekswesen* 5 (1888): 118–119.

35. One such manuscript is Cpl. 1158, which dates from the twelfth century and contains the *Viaticus peregrinantis* of Constantinus Africanus. The manuscript contains sixty-eight folios, and on the verso side of the last folio a hippopathological remedy has been added in the upper margin; the remedy is actually an incantation in Old High German! See Bartsch, 194; Schuba, *Die medizinischen Handschriften*, 116–117.

36. Bartsch, 47.

37. Bartsch, 55–56.

38. Elmar Mittler, "Bibliothek und Universität. Skizzen zu ihrer Wechselbeziehung," *Semper apertus*, Band IV, 8.

39. See Gerhard Eis, "Pferderezepte von Pfalzgraf Philipp dem Aufrichtigen," in his *Forschungen zur Fachprosa. Ausgewählte Beiträge* (Bern and Munich: Francke, 1971) 158–161.

40. Gundolf Keil, "Ludwig V., Pfalzgraf bei Rhein," in *Die deutsche Literatur des Mittelalters. Verfasserlexikon*, ed. Kurt Ruh, 2nd ed. (Berlin and New York: de Gruyter, 1985), vol. 5, cols. 1028–1029.

41. Gerhard Eis, "Heinrich Münsingers 'Regimen sanitatis in fluxu catarrhali ad pectus,'" in his *Forschungen zur Fachprosa*, 81–90.

42. Colette Jeudy and Ludwig Schuba, "Erhard Knab und die Heidelberger Universität im Spiegel von Handschriften und Akteneinträgen," *Quellen und Forschungen aus italienischen Archiven und Bibliotheken* 61 (1981): 90.

43. Hellmut Salowsky, "Das zwölfbändige 'Buch der Medizin' zu Heidelberg. Ein Autograph Kurfürst Ludwigs V.," *Heidelberger Jahrbücher* 17 (1973): 40.

44. "Otto Heinrich, Kurfürst von der Pfalz," in *Allgemeine Deutsche Biographie* (1887; Berlin: Duncker & Humblot, 1970), vol. 24, 719.

45. The electors preserved some of the commissioned works in their personal library, which was not always in Heidelberg castle. As the fortunes of the Palatine electors declined after Otto Heinrich, some of these holdings were sold or moved to other residences. Hence, several of the manuscripts cited here are now part of other collections. Knab's pharmacopoeia, called the *Heidelberger Pharmakopöe*, is in the Karlsruhe Generallandesarchiv, Pfälzer Kopialbuch, vol. 812. Münsinger's *Regimen sanitatis* is in the Bayerische Staatsbibliothek (Clm. 224, 212r–217r), as is Ludwig VI's *Diätbuch* (Cod. bav. 1544). However, there is an *Arzneibuch* in Heidelberg, Cpg. 193, which contains "Gutachten und Diätvorschriften für Kurf. Ludwig," prepared by Doctor Krauß in 1561, before Ludwig became elector.

46. I am currently completing work on an edition of the incantations found in the *Zwölfbändiges Buch der Medizin* and an examination of the relationship between medicine, magic, and religion in late medieval Germany as exemplified by Ludwig V's collection of medical manuscripts.

47. Lynn Thorndike provides a general introduction to Paracelsus's accomplishments and describes his influence in *A History of Magic and Experimental Science, Volume V: The Sixteenth Century* (New York and London: Columbia University Press, 1941) 616–651.

48. In "Kilian, Ottheinrich und Paracelsus," *Heidelberger Jahrbücher* 18 (1974): 37, Joachim Telle notes that Johannes Huser's edition of the works of Theophrastus von Hohenheim, the first extensive edition, prepared in 1589 with the support of the elector of Bavaria and the archbishop of Cologne, relied heavily on the Neuburg Paracelsian manuscript collection.

49. Karl Schottenloher, "Pfalzgraf Ottheinrich und Alexander von Suchten," *Zeitschrift für die Geschichte des Oberrheins*, n.s. 41 (1928): 603; and G.F. Hartlaub, "Die Kunst und das magische Weltbild" in *Ottheinrich. Gedenkschrift zur 400jährigen Wiederkehr seiner Kurfürstenzeit in der Pfalz (1556–1559)*, Ruperto-Carola. Sonderband, ed. Georg Poensgen (Heidelberg: Universität Heidelberg, 1956) 276.

50. Wille provides a description of Cpg. 467 and Cpg. 801, and Mittler discusses the *Alchimia opuscula* in *Bibliotheca Palatina*, 209–210.

Telle offers an extensive list of Otto Heinrich's alchemical manuscripts in "Kilian, Ottheinrich und Paracelsus," 41–42.

51. Bruce T. Moran, "Patronage and Institutions: Courts, Universities, and Academies in Germany; an Overview: 1550–1750," in *Patronage and Institutions. Science, Technology, and Medicine at the European Court 1500–1750*, ed. Bruce T. Moran (Rochester, NY: Boydell Press, 1991) 175.

52. Moran, 175.

53. Joachim Telle, "Kilian, Ottheinrich und Paracelsus," 41.

54. See Moran, 169–183. For a detailed examination of this question, see Bruce T. Moran, *The Alchemical World of the German Court. Occult Philosophy and Chemical Medicine in the Circle of Moritz of Hessen (1572–1632), Sudhoffs Archiv* Beiheft 29 (Stuttgart: Franz Steiner, 1991).

55. Viktor Fossel, "Aus den medizinischen Briefen des pfalzgräflichen Leibarztes Johannes Lange 1485–1565," *Sudhoffs Archiv* 7 (1913–1914): 238–252.

56. Mittler, *Bibliotheca Palatina*, 99.

57. Allen G. Debus, *The Chemical Philosophy. Paracelsian Science and Medicine in the Sixteenth and Seventeenth Centuries*, Vol. I (New York: Science History Publications [Neale Watson Academic Publications], 1977) 132.

58. Mittler, *Bibliotheca Palatina*, 106.

59. Wilhelm Doerr, "Der anatomische Gedanke und die Heidelberger Medizin," *Semper apertus*, Band IV, 120.

60. Rosemarie Jansen and Hans Helmut Jansen, "Die Pest in Heidelberg," *Semper apertus*, Band I, 376.

61. For a list of such works, see Jansen and Jansen, 378–381.

62. Schuba, "Die medizinische Fakultät im 15. Jahrhundert," 166–167, and Schuba, *Die medizinischen Handschriften*, 192–196.

# Multitudes of Middle English Medical Manuscripts, or the Englishing of Science and Medicine

*Linda Ehrsam Voigts*

The translation into Latin of Greek and Arabic texts has been widely regarded as a significant and beneficial event in the history of medieval Western science and medicine. The subsequent translation of many of these same texts into vernacular languages has, however, been largely neglected by scholarship. This neglect notwithstanding, the vernacularization—or laicization, or popularization—of scientific and medical writings is likewise a significant event that should be studied and understood in its own right.[1]

One approach to such a study is to focus on a specific country. My focus is on medieval England, which is in many ways typical of Europe as a whole, for every European country with university learning produced a considerable number of learned scientific and medical writings in its vernacular by 1500. England differs somewhat, however, owing to changes in linguistic hegemony. In most Continental countries, vernacular scientific and medical writing can be traced from the eleventh century and came into its own in the thirteenth or fourteenth centuries. In England, however, it appears to have begun in the late ninth century with the Alfredian reforms, and to have expanded by the time of the Conquest to some two hundred texts, including some half-dozen lengthy medical treatises and many short computistical writings. This development came to naught, however, with the Norman Conquest of 1066. After the Conquest, vernacular scientific and medical texts did not reappear in England until the thirteenth century, and then in Anglo-Norman. In the mid-fourteenth century, English-language texts began to reappear, and in the last third or quarter of the 1300s eclipsed Anglo-Norman texts.

In these last decades of the fourteenth century, English-language remedy books were joined by serious reworkings in English of Latin texts and Middle English writings of some originality, as in the examples of the anonymous 1392 Surgery,[2] Henry Daniel's compendious *Liber Uricrisiarum*,[3] the Englishing of the writings of the surgeon John of Arderne,[4] and, of course, Chaucer's *Treatise on the Astrolabe* and—what may well be—his *Equatorie of Planetis*.[5] These efforts represent the first movement in what became a groundswell of Englishing in the fifteenth century.

None of these late fourteenth-century figures—whether we call them translators or organizers or commentators—could know with any certainty that he was in the vanguard of a large movement, although there was precedent for vernacular texts on the Continent; the patronage of French texts at the Court of Charles V is a prominent example.[6] It is not surprising that many of the fourteenth- and early fifteenth-century Middle English texts indicate the tentative status of vernacularization in that they begin with a prologue defending the effort, sometimes with rubrics referring to the use of the "lingua materna."[7] Chaucer's prologue is, of course, the best known:

> And Lowys, yf so be that I shewe the in my lighte Englissh as trewe conclusions touching this mater, and not oonly as trewe but as many and as subtile conclusiouns, as ben shewid in Latyn in eny commune tretys of the Astrelabie, konne me the more thank. And preie God save the king, that is lord of this langage, and alle that him feith berith and obeieth, everich in his degre, the more and the lasse. But considre wel that I ne usurpe not to have founden this werk of my labour or of myn engyn. I n'am but a lewd compilator of the labour of olde astrologiens, and have it translatid in myn Englissh oonly for thy doctrine. And with this swerd shal I sleen envie.

> [And Lewis, if it is that I show you in my easy English conclusions to be true concerning this matter, and not only that they are true but also that the conclusions are as manifold and as subtle as those that are demonstrated in Latin in any ordinary treatise on the astrolabe, you can thank me the more. So too, pray that God save the King, who is lord of this language, and all those who are loyal to him and obey him, each in his degree, greater and less. But know well that I do not claim to have created this treatise by my own labor or from my own ingenuity. I am only a vernacular compiler of the work of old astrologers and have translated it into my English solely for your teaching. And with this sword shall I slay envy.][8]

Chaucer need not have been defensive, however, for the *Treatise on the Astrolabe* was part of a trickle that became a flood tide in fifteenth-century England. This phenomenon of the vernacularization of thousands of scientific and medical texts in late medieval England has long deserved study,[9] but the neglect of fifteenth-century Middle English texts can be at least partially understood because the large majority of these texts remain unidentified in infrequently consulted fifteenth-century manuscripts.

In contrast, Latin medieval treatises have been much more accessible. Historians of science and medicine know that the single most important research tool for the study of medieval science is the *Catalogue of Incipits of Mediaeval Scientific Writings in Latin* by Lynn Thorndike and Pearl Kibre—often cited with some affection as *TK*.[10] *TK* is a magnum opus that represents the larger part of a lifetime of collaborative effort on the part of these two scholars. There has never been a comparable tool, however, to provide access to the scientific and medical writings in the vernacular languages of medieval Europe. Nor, in any instance, has the entire body of scientific writing in any medieval vernacular been comprehensively studied. Most work has been done on Anglo-Norman (almost singlehandedly by Tony Hunt in several books and a dozen articles)[11] and in the study of German *Fachprosa* in the tradition represented by scholars at Würzburg such as Gundolf Keil and Bernhard Schnell, but many vernacular scientific texts remain unstudied, and many remain unidentified.

In my own work with Old English (OE) and Middle English (ME) medical writing, I became over the years more and more aware of the difficulty of ascertaining the manuscript witnesses to these texts. My experience with a ME version of a university treatise on theoretical phlebotomy is typical. A ten years' search for manuscript witnesses uncovered two manuscripts containing independent translations. Michael McVaugh and I published editions of both and a comparative analysis of the two texts, and five years later, in the course of research on the Voigts-Kurtz database, I found in an uncatalogued manuscript another redaction of the longer version.[12]

Still another example of a textual problem caused by lack of information can be seen in the recently published edition and study of the ME anesthetic *dwale*.[13] After I established the text on the basis of twenty-seven manuscripts, four additional manuscripts came to our attention. Likewise, in spite of many years' labor by Margaret Ogden and Björn Wallner on the manuscripts containing the ME Guy de Chauliac, another manuscript, an uncatalogued Jesus College, Cambridge, codex containing the only complete text of the third and fullest ME version of that surgery, has recently come to light.[14]

This lack of access is a much greater problem for Middle English than for Old English texts. Among the surviving tenth- and eleventh-century OE writings—all of which appear to have been identified—we have recorded 199 texts in our database that are scientific and medical; all of these were edited in the nineteenth or twentieth century, and most of them have been studied in some detail.

The situation is, however, very different for Middle English. Scarcely any scientific or medical texts survive from the *early* part of the period, because of the linguistic hegemony of Latin and Anglo-Norman after the Conquest. However, from the period 1350 to 1500, English reasserted itself, and virtually thousands of surviving English vernacular scientific and medical texts were written, the vast majority of them unstudied, most of them unidentified, and many of them uncatalogued or inadequately catalogued.

Since 1985, Patricia Deery Kurtz and I have attempted to remedy this situation, to produce a companion to Thorndike-Kibre for the English medieval vernacular—a *VK* to complement *TK*. There will be two end products of this project. The first is a database in ASCII format, now essentially complete with information on approximately 7,700 OE and ME texts, which we hope to make available in CD-ROM format. The second product will be a companion volume for the English vernacular to Thorndike-Kibre, although it will differ from it in two respects: in specifying individual entry numbers, and in providing six specialized indices.[15]

Because prologues and texts often have textual histories independent of one another, it was necessary to enter information on them in the database separately. The same ME text may be found with or without a prologue, or with differing prologues in different manuscripts, and the same prologue can introduce different texts. The database must of necessity provide cross-references between prologues and texts. It must also provide cross-references between Latin incipit and the first words in English when a ME text begins in Latin.

It was possible to begin data entry for *VK* in some cases with information from recent detailed manuscript catalogues and from Index of Middle English Prose handlists, which must, of course, be supplemented for verse texts. However, it proved necessary to obtain most data from the surviving medieval manuscripts. For each manuscript witness to a text or prologue, we have entered in the database the incipit and information on author, English and Latin titles, translator, manuscript, subject categories, and bibliographical citations. We have tried, wherever possible, to indicate "embedded texts" within compendia, but we cannot claim to have caught them all. There will be tasks for our successors.

The much smaller Old English section of two hundred entries is coded to distinguish it from Middle English for linguistic and orthographic reasons, as well as for the fact that three centuries separate OE from ME texts. All OE entries appear at the beginning of the conflation and can be distinguished from ME citations in the indices.

For Old English, the incipit is recorded in the orthography of the standard published edition; for Middle English, modern orthography is used for those words that survive into Modern English, and the headword spelling of the *Middle English Dictionary* is used for those words that do not survive. We attempt to modernize spelling without modernizing language, admittedly a difficult distinction. Although there are important arguments against modernizing, we chose modern orthography because it resolves problems of determining the priority of manuscript witnesses, it eliminates problems of alphabetical order, it makes the texts accessible to historians of science and medicine without extensive linguistic training, and it makes computer conflation of identical incipits possible.

We now have in the database records for approximately 7,700 witnesses to texts, of which two hundred are Old English and the rest Middle English. We trust that sheer numbers, if nothing else, will give the lie to the myth that the medieval scientific and medical writings of England are mostly Latin.[16]

An overview of the proportions of data in the Catalogue of Scientific and Medical Writings in Old and Middle English in the present database may provide a sense of the topography of the vast body of ME scientific and medical writing. Such a survey can be accomoplished by an analysis of the six indices that provide access to the conflated incipits with bibliographical citation. The six indices provide access to text records headed by incipit through author, title, translator, Thorndike-Kibre equivalence, manuscript, and subject fields.

The index for Thorndike-Kibre correspondences is fairly straightforward, although it has proved necessary to indicate a one-to-one *VK* to *TK* entry correspondence by assigning letters of the alphabet, exclusive of O, to each *TK* column. A *VK* entry may have more than one *TK* citation as in the case of the ME version of a poem on the four humors, where *TK* lists the Latin text under both "Sanguineus . . ." and "Largeus. . . ."

The second of the two shorter indices is the Translator Index. This Index will never be extensive, as it is uncommon for translators to be identified, but it is of interest, not least because some hitherto unknown names of English translators—beyond the familiar Henry Daniel, John Lelamour, and John Metham—

are John Raynar, John Higins, and a translator designated "Brokhole."

One of the indices that will be useful to those interested in the vernacularization of specific Latin texts is the Author Index. It must, however, be used with care because, first, we have by no means identified many authors of unattributed texts; second, prologue entries inflate the numbers for particular authors like Chaucer (in the case of the *Treatise on the Astrolabe*); and third, we cannot claim to have recognized every spurious attribution and tagged that text with an asterisk. We only hope that our effort to differentiate between authentic and attributed texts—however incomplete—represents an improvement on Thorndike-Kibre.

The Author Index makes clear that the fifteen authors or attributed authors whose names appear most frequently with ME scientific and medical texts are as follows:

1. George Ripley
2. Ramon Lull (spurious alchemical attributions)
3. Geoffrey Chaucer
4. John of Burgundy
5. John of Arderne
6. Macer
7. Gilbertus Anglicus; it should be noted that this reckoning does not include all the gynecology texts that Monica Green has identified as deriving from the *Compendium*, and one should note that when those are included, it is clear that Gilbertus was extremely popular in fifteenth-century English versions, far more so than in Latin versions of preceding centuries[17]
8. Albertus Magnus (primarily spurious alchemical attributions)
9. Galen
10. Guy de Chauliac
11. Lanfranc
12. Roger Bacon (primarily spurious alchemical attributions)
13. Hippocrates
14. Thomas Norton
15. Arnald of Villanova (primarily spurious alchemical attributions)

It is, however, true that many of the most interesting ME texts seem not to have circulated widely. Those which survive in only a few copies include, for example, the ME versions of texts by or attributed to Abraham ibn Ezra, Benevenutus Grassus/Grapheus, Bernard of Gordon, Hunayn ibn Ishaq, John of Gaddesden, John of Rupescissa, Peter of Spain, Regiomontanus, Richard of Wallingford, Roger of Hereford, Theodoric of Lucca, and Zael, to name only a few; John North, for example, cites Richard of Wallingford's *Exafrenon* as the only text by that author to be Englished,[18] but the *Declarationes* was also translated into the vernacular, and in fact, survives in three separate ME translations.[19]

Not surprisingly, treatises popular in the vernacular circulated without attribution to any author. According to our Title Index, the most popular of these appears to have been the herbal that circulated under the rubric, "Here Men May See the Virtues of Herbs."[20] We have so far recorded more than forty instances of this text that appears to derive ultimately from Macer but is not to be confused with the Middle English translation of the traditional *De Viribus (or Virtutibus) Herbarum*.[21]

Nearly as popular as "Here Men May See the Virtues of Herbs" was the herbal *Agnus Castus* (ca. thirty instances)[22] and the *Wise Book of Astronomy and Philosophy* (also ca. 30 entries).[23] Three other, somewhat less popular, anonymous texts—all of which deserve good modern editions—were the *Virtues of Rosemary* (ca. fifteen texts), the *Liber Uricrisiarum* (ca. fifteen copies),[24] and the *Virtues of Betony* (ca. twelve copies).

Although the Title Index is useful for identifying popular texts not attributed to authors, many popular ME texts are both unattributed and untitled. Indeed, the regimen of health that usually begins with some version of "In January drink white wine fasting and bloodletting forbear . . ." survives in many manuscripts and merits study, as does the larger question of the popularity of vernacular regimen of health treatises.[25]

The number of surviving manuscripts containing vernacular English science and medicine is considerable, as the database establishes. The Manuscript Index at present cites ca. eight hundred manuscripts. We hope that the *VK* manuscript index will be an improvement on *TK* (which does not index manuscripts), in that it will enable the reader to determine what ME texts occur in the same codex. It will not, however, allow the user to ascertain what texts in other languages occur in the same codex.

Some manuscript collections are particularly rich in codices containing ME scientific and medical texts. In some instances, such as the Sloane, Ashmole, and Wellcome collections, the incidence of these texts is not surprising, for the collectors were primarily interested in assembling libraries of scientific and medical writings. There are ten collections which have more than twenty-five manuscripts represented in the *VK* database:

1. The British Library Collection assembled by Sir Hans Sloane (the largest collection by far)—241
2. The Collection in the Bodleian Library assembled by Elias Ashmole—64
3. Trinity College Cambridge—63
4. The Harley Collection in the British Library—54
5. The Rawlinson Collection in the Bodleian Library—41
6. Wellcome Historical Medical Library (a collection begun by Sir Henry Wellcome)—29
7. The Royal Collection in the British Library—28
8. Cambridge University Library—27
9. The Additional Collection in the British Library—26
10. The Bodley Collection in the Bodleian Library—26

The largest of the *VK* indices is the Subject Index. It provides proportional information on the most popular subject fields, even when based not on raw data, but on preliminary conflation. Each of twenty-five categories occurs at least fifty times in our subject indices. It should be noted that any given text may be entered with several subject fields. The largest category, *Recipes*, deserves some explanation. Only in exceptional circumstances does *VK* record a single recipe; our citations are to collections of recipes, indicating the number of recipes in a collection. We define a collection arbitrarily as a minimum of three recipes in the same hand, and "Recipes" are in fact subdivided into twenty subcategories in the Subject Index.

The following list indicating the approximate number of citations in our subject fields provides an overview of proportional representation:

| | | |
|---|---|---|
| 1. | Recipes | over 2,500 |
| 2. | Alchemy | 1,000 |
| 3. | Herbs and Herbal Medicine | 375 |
| 4. | Urine and Uroscopy | 350 |
| 5. | Bloodletting | 300 |
| 6. | Charms | 300 |
| 7. | Prognostication | 275 |
| 8. | Zodiac and Signs of | 250 |
| 9. | Planet and Planets | 225 |
| 10. | Astrology | 225 |
| 11. | Lucky and Unlucky Days | 200 |
| 12. | Humors | 200 |
| 13. | Regimen of Health | 175 |
| 14. | Astronomy | 175 |
| 15. | Moon | 175 |
| 16. | Plague | 125 |
| 17. | Etiology | 100 |
| 18. | Gynecology and Obstetrics | 100 |
| 19. | Surgery | 100 |
| 20. | Diet | 100 |
| 21. | Measure and Measurement, and Weights and Measures | 75 |
| 22. | Horse | 75 |
| 23. | Equine medicine | 75 |
| 24. | Physiognomy | 75 |
| 25. | Philosophers' Stone | 75 |

Thousands of scientific and medical texts were translated or composed in the English vernacular in the fourteenth and fifteenth centuries, and considerable numbers of them survive. These deserve study in the aggregate for what they tell us about the era (Why, for example, does alchemy appear to loom larger in vernacular treatises than in Latin writings?). They deserve analysis as groups of related texts (What role did the vernacular regimen of health treatise play in popularizing academic medicine?), and many hitherto neglected individual texts, such as the ME version(s) of the *Antidotarium Nicolai*, merit study in their own right. Patricia Deery Kurtz and I hope that our Catalogue of Incipits of Scientific and Medical Writings in Old and Middle English—both in electronic and book form—will provide a tool valuable to the study of medieval science and medicine. In identifying, classifying, and locating the scientific and medical texts in the English vernacular that survive from the fourteenth and fifteenth centuries it will, we hope, facilitate the study of the late-medieval Englishing of science and medicine.

## NOTES

1. On the importance of the translation of Greek and Arabic texts into Latin, see, e.g., chapter 9, "The Revival of Learning in the West," and chapter 10, "The Recovery and Assimilation of Greek and Islamic Science," in David C. Lindberg, *The Beginnings of Western Science* (Chicago: University of Chicago Press, 1992), and Chapter 1, "The Formation of Western European Medicine," in Nancy G. Siraisi, *Medieval and Early Renaissance Medicine* (Chicago: University of Chicago Press, 1990). One of the few historians of science to comment, even briefly, on vernacularization is John North in "Astronomy and Mathematics," in *The History of the University of Oxford*, Vol. II, Late Medieval Oxford, ed. J. I. Catto and Ralph Evans (Oxford: Clarendon Press, 1992) 173.

2. Richard Grothé, "Le ms. Wellcome 564: deux traités de chirurgie en moyen-anglais," Ph.D. diss., Université de Montréal, 1984. Dr. Grothé is preparing an edition of these two surgeries for publication.

3. Joanne Jasin, "A Critical Edition of the Middle English *Liber Uricrisiarum* in Wellcome MS 225," Ph.D. diss., Tulane University, 1983. See also the discussion of this work by Ralph Hanna III in "Henry Daniel's *Liber Uricrisiarum*, Book I, Chapters 1–3," in *Popular and Practical Science of Medieval England*, ed. Lister Matheson (East Lansing, MI: Colleagues Press, 1994) 185–218.

4. See, e.g., Peter Murray Jones, "Four Middle English Translations of John of Arderne," in *Latin and Vernacular: Studies in Late-*

*Medieval Texts and Manuscripts*, ed. A.J. Minnis (Cambridge: D.S. Brewer, 1989) 61–89.

5. *A Treatise on the Astrolabe* in *The Riverside Chaucer*, ed. Larry D. Benson (Boston: Houghton Mifflin, 1987) 662–683, and *The Equatorie of Planetis*, ed. Derek J. Price (Cambridge: Cambridge University Press, 1955). John North argues in favor of Chaucer's authorship of the *Equatorie* in his *Chaucer's Universe* (Oxford: Clarendon Press, 1988), whereas Kari Anne Rand-Schmidt, *The Authorship of The Equatorie of the Planetis* (Cambridge: D.S. Brewer, 1993), argues against it.

6. See, e.g., Peter F. Dembowski, "Learned Latin Treatises in French: Inspiration, Plagiarism, and Translation," *Viator* 17 (1985): 255–269.

7. See, e.g., the prologue (pp. 37–39) to a lengthy learned medical treatise (39–228; atelous) in Cambridge, Gonville and Caius College MS. 176/97, discussed in Linda E. Voigts and Michael R. McVaugh, eds., *A Latin Technical Phlebotomy and Its Middle English Translation*, Transactions of the American Philosophical Society 74 (Philadelphia, 1984) 14–15. The Prologue is also to be found in Cambridge, Trinity College MS. R.14.52, ff. 159–160.

8. *The Riverside Chaucer*, 662, ll. 50–64.

9. One of the first studies to begin to address the vast numbers of ME treatises was Rossell Hope Robbins, "Medical Manuscripts in Middle English," *Speculum* 45 (1970): 393–415, but Robbins underestimated the number of surviving texts and manuscripts.

10. Rev. ed. (Cambridge, MA: Medieval Academy of America, 1963).

11. See, e.g, Hunt's *Popular Medicine in Thirteenth-Century England: Introduction and Texts* (Cambridge: D.S. Brewer, 1990).

12. Voigts and McVaugh (see n. 7) edited the longer version from Cambridge, Gonville and Caius MS. 176/97, pp. 1–11, and the shorter (App. A) from Cambridge, Gonville and Caius MS. 176/97, pp. 205–206. Another version can be found in British Library Sloane MS. 3217, ff. 119v–125v.

13. Linda E. Voigts and Robert P. Hudson, "A drynke that men callen dwale to make a man to slepe whyle men kerven hem: A Surgical Anesthetic from Late Medieval England," in *Health, Disease and Healing in Medieval Culture*, ed. Sheila Campbell, Bert Hall, and David Klausner (New York: St. Martin's Press, 1992) 34–56.

14. On Cambridge, Jesus College MS Q.G.23, see Björn Wallner, "A Newly Discovered Guy de Chauliac Manuscript," *Notes and Queries* 236, n.s. 38 (1991): 159.

15. We have been fortunate to have support for this study from a three-year grant from the Reference Materials Program of the National Endowment for the Humanities.

16. The database is stored in ASCII format. We manipulate it on a VAX-VMS mainframe with two programs in C-language written by Michael Fatino and Barry Archer. These programs alphabetize the data, conflate identical incipits, and produce the six indices.

17. Monica H. Green, "Obstetrical and Gynecological Texts in Middle English," *Studies in the Age of Chaucer* 14 (1992): 53–88. Faye M. Getz identified the ME translation of the *Compendium Medicinae* of Gilbertus Anglicus and edited the version in Wellcome Historical Medical Library MS. 537 in *Healing and Society in Medieval England: A Middle English Translation of the Pharmaceutical Writings of Gilbertus Anglicus* (Madison: University of Wisconsin Press, 1991).

18. *Richard of Wallingford: An Edition of His Writings*, 3 vols. (Oxford: Clarendon Press, 1976).

19. I am preparing an edition of the ME versions of the *Declarationes*.

20. Pol Grymonprez, ed., *"Here Men May Se the Vertues off Herbes,"* Scripta 3 (Brussels, 1981), is an edition of the version in Bodleian Bodley MS. 483.

21. Gösta Frisk, ed., *A Middle English Translation of Macer Floridus "De Viribus Herbarum,"* Essays and Studies on English Language and Literature 3 (Upsala, 1949), is an edition of the version in Stockholm, Royal Library MS. X.91.

22. Gösta Brodin, ed., *Agnus Castus: A Middle English Herbal*, Essays and Studies on English Language and Literature 6 (Upsala, 1950) draws on most, but by no means all, of the manuscripts.

23. Jeanne Krochalis and Edward Peters, eds. *The World of Piers Plowman* (Philadelphia: University of Pennsylvania Press, 1975), 3–17 and 218–228, is an edition of the version in Cambridge University Library MS. Ll.4.14. See also Paul Acker, "The Missing Conclusion of *The Book of Physiognomy*," *Medium Ævum* 54 (1985): 266–270.

24. See n. 3.

25. W.L. Braekman, ed., *Studies on Alchemy, Diet, Medecine [sic] and Prognostication in Middle English*, Scripta 22 (Brussels, 1988 for 1986) 58–60, is an edition of the version in British Library Sloane MS. 962.

# Contributors

**Melitta Weiss Adamson** studied German literature at the University of Vienna, Austria, the University of Waterloo, and the University of Toronto. She is currently Assistant Professor of German and Assistant Professor of History of Medicine at The University of Western Ontario. Her dissertation, *Food and Drink in Medical-Dietetic Fachliteratur from 1050 to 1400* (Toronto, 1989) and M.A. thesis, *Zur Entstehung, Tradierung und Lexik deutscher Kochbücher und Rezepte des Spätmittelalters,* (Waterloo, 1983) laid the foundation for publications on dietetics, Hildegard's *Physica,* pregnancy regimens, and humor in medieval Fachliteratur. A book of essays on *Food in the Middle Ages,* to be published by Garland, is in preparation.

**William C. Crossgrove** took his A.B. in German at Ohio University in 1959. He received his Ph.D. in Germanic Linguistics at the University of Texas at Austin in 1962 and subsequently joined the faculty of Brown University, where he has served two terms as Chair of the German Department and is currently Professor of German and Comparative Literature. His research in recent years has focused on medieval German herbals and other nonliterary texts.

**Peter Murray Jones** is Fellow and Librarian at King's College, Cambridge. He is the author of *Medieval Medical Miniatures* (London/University of Texas, 1984) and "Medical Books Before the Invention of Printing" in *Thornton's Medical Books, Libraries and Collectors* (1990). In addition, he has worked on the manuscript tradition of the texts of the fourteenth-century English surgeon John of Arderne and has published studies on both the Latin and the English-language manuscripts in that tradition. He is currently writing a book on sickness and healing in the Middle Ages.

**Gundolf Keil** received his Ph.D. at Heidelberg in 1961, his M.D. at Bonn in 1969, and his Dr. med. habil. at Freiburg in 1970. He currently holds the Chair in the History of Medicine at the University of Würzburg, where he directs the Institute for the History of Medicine. His publications focus primarily on medieval German medical texts, although he has also written on ancient and modern medicine. He is editor of the journal *Sudhoffs Archiv* and coeditor of *Die Deutsche Literatur des Mittelalters: Verfasserlexikon* (second edition) as well as *Lexikon des Mittelalters.* Through the numerous volumes he has edited and coedited, along with the journal *Würzburger medizinhistorische Mitteilungen* and the monograph series *Würzburger medizinhistorische Forschungen,* his impact on the study of medieval medicine goes even beyond his own numerous and influential publications.

**John M. Riddle** received his Ph.D. in History from the University of North Carolina, Chapel Hill and held a Fulbright postdoctoral fellowship at the History of Medicine Institute in Bonn, Germany. He is currently Professor of History at North Carolina State University. He is the author of five books: *Marbode of Rennes' De lapidibus* (1977); "Dioscorides" in the series, *Catalogus Translationum et Commentariorum* (1980); *Dioscorides on Pharmacy and Medicine* (1985), for which he received the Urdang Medal; *Contraception and Abortion from the Ancient World to the Renaissance* (1992); and *Quid pro quo: Studies in the History of Drugs* (1992).

**Bernhard Schnell** studied German literature, history, and social sciences at the Ludwig-Maximilians-Universität München, where he received his doctorate with a dissertation on *Thomas Peuntner 'Büchlein von der Liebhabung Gottes'* (a revised version was published in the series *Münchener Texte und Untersuchungen* in 1984). He is the lead editor of *Vocabularius Ex quo. Überlieferungsgeschichtliche Ausgabe*

(Tübingen 1988–89), a five volume critical edition of the most important late medieval Latin-German glossary. In addition to numerous articles, lectures, and book reviews (including especially detailed reviews of manuscript catalogues), he completed his "Habilitation" in the history of medicine in 1989 with a pioneering study of medieval German medicinal herbals. He currently teaches in the Institute for the History of Medicine, University of Würzburg.

**Debra L. Stoudt** earned her Ph.D. in German at the University of North Carolina, Chapel Hill. She is presently Associate Professor of German at the University of Toledo (Toledo, Ohio). She has received grants from the DAAD, the Fulbright Commission, the National Endowment for the Humanities, the Germanistic Society of America, and the University of Toledo. She has published articles on the letters and sermons of the German mystics and she is currently working on a monograph on the *Twelve Books of Medicine* of Ludwig V of Heidelberg.

**Linda Ehrsam Voigts** is Curators' Professor of English at the University of Missouri-Kansas City. She is the author of *A Handlist of Middle English in Harvard Manuscripts* (1985) and coauthor of *A Latin Technical Phlebotomy and Its Middle English Translation* (1984), as well as numerous major articles and chapters of books.

**Faith Wallis** holds a joint appointment in the Department of History and the Department of Social Studies of Medicine at McGill University. Her published work focuses on the medieval *computus*, and on scientific and medical manuscripts. She is currently working on a comprehensive study of *computus*.

# Index of Manuscripts

# Index